THE ANTI-INFLAMMATORY DIET COOKBOOK

More Than 150 Recipes for Instant, Overnight, Meal-Prepped, and Easy Comfort Foods

Marco Williams

TABLE OF CONTENTS

DESSERT RECIPES

INTRODUCTION

Anti-inflammatory diet is a term used to describe a diet that limits the intake of meats, refined grains, and sugars and emphasizes dietary plant products. The theory is that dietary choices can impact the body's inflammatory response to injury or stress. A dietary pattern low in saturated fat and high in fruits, vegetables, legumes, and whole grains may significantly reduce risk of inflammation-related diseases including cardiovascular disease, cancer, and autoimmune disorders.

An anti-inflammatory diet is generally based on the Mediterranean diet and the DASH diet, and in some cases the new Nordic diet.

It can be modified for individual needs, such as vegetarian or vegan diets.

An anti-inflammatory diet may aid the treatment of a number of diseases, including anxiety disorder, atherosclerosis, cancer, chronic obstructive pulmonary disease, autoimmune disorders, multiple sclerosis, allergies, infectious disease, viral disease, hypertension, rheumatoid arthritis, inflammatory bowel disease, and chronic pain. Several studies have found an inverse association between higher detailed inflammatory response and the amount of whole grain in the diet. Whole grains, peas, green pasture, pansy, and beans support bone health and preserve bone strength.

While no nutrition interventions have been confirmed to reduce inflammation in situations like rheumatoid arthritis, research on the use of probiotics as a treatment for IBD suggests a positive effect of probiotic use on inflammatory markers.

An anti-inflammatory diet may limit total and LDL cholesterol levels, which may be beneficial. A diet high in anti-inflammatory components may help to reduce risk factors for chronic conditions, including asthma, cancer, and arthritis, via the manipulation of inflammatory cytokines.

A green, high plant-food diet is reliably associated with reduced inflammation high levels, whereas a high-fat, high-meat diet is specifically associated with increased inflammation levels.

The effect on inflammation of various dietary interventions is a current research topic and is the subject of several reviews. A high intake of saturated fatty acids (SFAs) – predominantly from animal sources – is connected with higher levels of inflammatory markers. This high intake is associated with cardiovascular disease. Plant oils (both olive oil and rapeseed oil) have an anti-inflammatory effect.

A high intake of carbohydrates (especially simple carbohydrates from sugars and refined grains) is linked with higher levels of inflammatory markers. This high intake is associated with an increased risk of diabetes, hypertension, obesity, and CVDs. The Mediterranean Diet is recommended for cardiovascular health and includes a high intake of legumes, fruit and vegetables, and a moderate intake of fish, whole grains, and olive oil. Other healthy diets that may have a reduced inflammatory potential include the alternative and the Nordic diet.

What Is Chronic Inflammation?

When you lose a body part, your body doesn't spend too much time mourning it - it's busy growing a new one. However, sometimes it's the loss of a healthy tissue that takes the body longer to overcome. Chronic inflammation is the chronic reaction to a chronic problem that is occurring in a tissue or part of the body.

Too much of a certain protein compound in the body, named interleukin-6, is released in the bloodstream of persons with chronic inflammation. Chronic inflammation reduces the body's immunities as well as decrease its ability to fight off foreign invasions.

More simply, chronic inflammation means that in a body tissue or organ some part of the tissue is being treated by the body as if it is a foreign invader to be attacked and destroyed. Inflammation also causes discomfort and pain. The body's response to injury is to seek to identify the chemical compounds that may have invaded the tissue, to sound the alarm to other parts of the body, and then to mobilize an inflammatory response to overcome the invading forces.

In the case of chronic inflammation, the inflammation is occurring after a period of time rather than occurring immediately and subsiding. Since the damage to the tissue becomes more severe, the tissue is no longer as able to function for its intended purpose, and the body must then shore up the impaired cells with a layer of scar tissue. This is why it is so difficult to heal from an injury that has become chronic.

Reasons for Chronic Inflammation

Chronic inflammation may be due to infections, such as tuberculosis, long term viral infections, or bacterial infections, also known as sepsis or septicemia. Parasites in the bowel, or even lactose intolerance, can also lead to chronic inflammation. More issues like clogged blood vessels and autoimmune diseases can also contribute.

When a cause cannot be determined, but the inflammation continues and causes pain and other issues increasing in severity, the condition may be called idiopathic inflammation. Sometimes, the root problem itself may be difficult to determine, as the body has no known foreign invader. For this reason, medication may be given to suppress the inflammatory response, as the medications can then attack the cause more directly than trying to stop the symptoms of inflammation, which is a different matter.

Best Ways to Address Chronic Inflammation

Because chronic inflammation is a recurring and recurring problem, diet and supplements are appropriate.

1. Reduce Saturated Fats and Protein Intake

There are many ways to reduce the intake of protein and fat in a person's diet. Simply avoiding red meat for muscle meats is not enough, for example, as chicken, turkey, veal, and fish also contain saturated fats. Cold-water fish, such as salmon and herring are better choices than the others.

2. Alcohol Consumption

Excessive alcohol consumption is a no-no for many reasons, but one of them is that it introduces additional saturated fats into the body.

3. Pasteurized Milk

Raw milk is a good source of healthy nutrients and also contains enzymes that have antioxidant effects. But pasteurizing milk destroys the enzymes, as well as some nutrients in milk, and changes the protein structures. This affects the protein that is absorbed by the body and causes problems.

4. Nuts and Legumes

These substances are, however, high in protein. The problem with soy and nuts is that the protein in these substances is not in the form of complete amino acids, so this protein cannot be absorbed completely by the body to make new tissues.

5. Polyunsaturated Oils

Olive oil and other monounsaturated oils are highly recommended for other reasons, but the polyunsaturated oils may actually be inducing oxidative stress and inducing inflammation, so they are best avoided.

A diet high in fruits and vegetables is good, but not if any of the vegetables are green, such as broccoli, spinach, or lettuce. Green vegetables, as should come as no surprise, have high levels of protein. Fruits, on the other hand, have very little protein, except for watermelon and guava, which is not too high.

Some forms of swelling or inflammation, such as those caused by injuries to tissue, are actually beneficial to the body. The signal needs for treatment and attract other components of the immune system to the site of the injury.

All in all, chronic inflammation is a big problem in the body and difficult to heal. It is also difficult to treat, requiring vigilance and a healthy diet to avoid additional inflammation. You may have to avoid meats and should avoid soy and raw milk to get the best results.

When you suffer from chronic inflammation, it's not always clear what the root cause is. Medical experts point to one thing, while another group of experts points to something entirely different.

Medication for this condition is also controversial and often yields unpleasant side effects. Moreover, drug companies don't make very good money on medications that only treat symptoms, so they tend to ignore them. Therefore, this cookbook was created to help you find a natural and complete alternative to popping pills on a daily basis. It does not matter if your inflammation is caused by an infection, overconsumption of dairy, or even stress -- you can find a remedy in these recipes that is natural, effective, and will not have side effects.

BREAKFAST RECIPES

1. Buckwheat Cinnamon and Ginger Granola

Preparation Time: 15 minutes

Cooking Time: 40 minutes

Servings: 5

INGREDIENTS:

- ¼ cup Chia seeds
- ½ Cup Coconut Flakes
- 1 ½ Cup mixed Raw nuts
- 2 cups of gluten-free oats
- 1 cup of buckwheat groats
- 2 tbsp nut butter
- 4 tbsp of coconut oil
- 1 cup of sunflower seeds
- ½ cup of pumpkin seeds
- 1 ½ - 2 inches piece of ginger
- 1 tsp Ground Cinnamon
- 1/3 cup of Rice Malt Syrup
- 4 tbsp of raw cacao powder – Optional

DIRECTIONS:

1. Preheat the oven up to 180C
2. Blitz the nuts in your food processor and quickly blitz to chop roughly. Put the chopped nuts in a bowl and add all the other dry ingredients that combine well— oats, coconut, cinnamon, buckwheat, seeds, and salt in a low heat saucepan, melt the coconut oil gently.
3. Add the cacao powder (if used) to the wet mixture and blend. Put the wet batter over the dry mix, then mix well to make sure that everything is coated. Move the mixture to a wide baking tray lined with grease-proof paper or coconut oil greased. Be sure to uniformly distribute the mixture for 35-40 minutes, turning the mixture halfway

through. Bake until the granola is fresh and golden!

4. Serve with your favorite nut milk, coconut yogurt scoop, fresh fruit, and superfoods—goji berries, flax seeds, bee pollen, whatever you like! Mix it up every single day.

NUTRITION: Calories: 220 Carbs: 38g Fat: 5g Protein: 7g

2. Fruity Flaxseed Breakfast Bowl

Preparation Time: 8 minutes

Cooking Time: 5 minutes

Servings: 1

INGREDIENTS:

For the Porridge:

- ¼-cup flaxseeds, freshly ground
- ¼-tsp cinnamon, ground
- 1-cup almond or coconut milk
- 1 medium banana, mashed
- A pinch of fine-grained sea salt

For the Toppings:

- Blueberries, fresh or defrosted
- Walnuts, chopped raw
- Pure maple syrup (optional)

DIRECTIONS:

1. In a medium-sized saucepan placed over medium heat, combine all the porridge ingredients. Stir constantly for 5 minutes, or until the porridge thickens and comes to a low boil.
2. Transfer the cooked porridge in a serving bowl. Garnish with the toppings and pour a bit of maple syrup if you want it a little sweeter.

NUTRITION: Calories: 780 Fat: 26g Protein: 39g Sodium: 270mg Total Carbs: 117.5g

3. Perky Paleo Potato & Protein Powder

Preparation Time: 8 minutes

Cooking Time: 0 minutes

Servings: 1

INGREDIENTS:

- 1 small sweet potato, pre-baked and fleshed out
- 1-Tbsp protein powder
- 1 small banana, sliced
- ¼-cup blueberries
- ¼-cup raspberries
- Choice of toppings: cacao nibs, chia seeds, hemp hearts, favorite nut/seed butter (optional)

DIRECTIONS:

1. In a small serving bowl, mash the sweet potato using a fork. Add the protein powder. Mix well until thoroughly combined.
2. Arrange the banana slices, blueberries, and raspberries on top of the mixture. Garnish with your desired toppings. You can relish this breakfast meal, either cold or warm.

NUTRITION: Calories: 302 Fat: 10g Protein: 15.3g Sodium: 65mg Total Carbs: 46.7g

4. Spicy Shakshuka

Preparation Time: 12 minutes

Cooking Time: 37 minutes

Servings: 4

INGREDIENTS:

- 2-Tbsps extra-virgin olive oil
- 1-bulb onion, minced
- 1 jalapeño, seeded and minced
- 2-cloves garlic, minced
- 1-lb spinach
- Salt and freshly ground black pepper
- ¾-tsp coriander
- 1-tsp dried cumin
- 2-Tbsps harissa paste
- ½-cup vegetable broth
- 8-pcs large eggs
- Red pepper flakes, for serving
- Cilantro, chopped for serving
- Parsley, chopped for serving

DIRECTIONS:

1. Preheat your oven to 350°F.
2. Heat the oil in an oven-safe skillet placed over medium heat. Stir in the onion and sauté for 5 minutes.
3. Add the jalapeño and garlic, and sauté for a minute, or until fragrant. Add in the spinach, and cook for 5 minutes, or until the leaves entirely wilt.
4. Season the mixture with salt and pepper, coriander, cumin, and harissa. Cook further for 1 minute.
5. Transfer the mixture to your food processor—puree to a thick consistency. Pour in the broth and puree further until achieving a smooth texture.
6. Clean and grease the same skillet with nonstick cooking spray. Pour the pureed mixture. By using a wooden spoon, form eight circular wells.
7. Crack each egg gently into the wells. Put the skillet in the oven—Bake for 25 minutes, or poaching the eggs until fully set.
8. To serve, sprinkle the shakshuka with red pepper flakes, cilantro, and parsley to taste.

NUTRITION: Calories: 251 Fat: 8.3g Protein: 12.5g Sodium: 165mg Total Carbs: 33.6g

5. Choco Chia Banana Bowl

Preparation Time: 4 hours & 5 minutes

Cooking Time: 0 minutes

Servings: 3

INGREDIENTS:

- ½-cup chia seeds
- 1 large banana, very ripe
- ½-tsp pure vanilla extract
- 2-cups almond milk, unsweetened
- 1-Tbsp cacao powder
- 2-Tbsps raw honey or maple syrup
- 2-Tbsps cacao nibs for mixing in
- 2-Tbsps chocolate chips for mixing in
- 1 large banana, sliced for mixing in

DIRECTIONS:

1. Combine the chia seeds and banana in a mixing bowl. By using a fork, mash the banana and mix well until thoroughly combined. Pour in the vanilla and almond milk. Whisk until no more lumps appear.
2. Pour half of the mix in a glass container, and cover it. Add the cacao and syrup to the remaining half mixture in the bowl. Mix well until fully incorporated. Pour this mixture in another glass container, and cover it. Chill for at least 4 hours.
3. To serve, layer the chilled chia puddings equally in three serving bowls. Alternate the layers with the ingredients for mixing-in.

NUTRITION: Calories: 293 Fat: 9.7g Protein: 14.6g Sodium: 35mg Total Carbs: 43.1g

6. Power Protein Porridge

Preparation Time: 15 minutes

Cooking Time: 8 minutes

Servings: 2

INGREDIENTS:

- ¼-cup walnut or pecan halves, roughly chopped
- ¼-cup toasted coconut, unsweetened
- 2-Tbsps hemp seeds
- 2-Tbsps whole chia seeds
- ¾-cup almond milk, unsweetened
- ¼-cup coconut milk
- ¼-cup almond butter, roasted
- ½-tsp turmeric, ground
- 1-Tbsp extra virgin coconut oil or MCT oil
- 2-Tbsps erythritol or 5-10 drops liquid stevia (optional)
- A pinch of ground black pepper
- ½-tsp cinnamon or ½-tsp vanilla powder

DIRECTIONS:

1. Put the walnuts, flaked coconut, and hemp seeds in a hot saucepan. Roast the mixture for 2 minutes, or until fragrant. Stir a few times to prevent burning. Transfer the roasted mix in a bowl. Set aside.
2. Combine the almond and coco milk in a small saucepan placed over medium heat. Heat the mixture.
3. After heating, but not boiling, switch off the heat. Add all the remaining ingredients. Mix well until thoroughly combined. Set aside for 10 minutes.
4. Combine half of the roasted mix with the porridge. Scoop the porridge into two serving bowls. Sprinkle each bowl with the remaining half of the roasted mixture and cinnamon powder. Serve the porridge immediately.

NUTRITION: Calories: 572 Fat: 19g Protein: 28.6g Sodium: 87mg Total Carbs: 81.5g Dietary Fiber: 10g

7. <u>Avo Toast with Egg</u>

Preparation Time: 15 minutes

Cooking Time: 0 minutes

Servings: 3

INGREDIENTS:

- 1½-tsp ghee
- 1-slice bread, gluten-free and toasted
- ½ avocado, thinly sliced
- A handful of spinach
- 1 egg scrambled or poached
- A sprinkle of red pepper flakes

DIRECTIONS:

1. Spread the ghee over the toasted bread. Top with the avocado slices and spinach leaves. Place a scrambled or poached egg on top. Finish off the garnishing with a sprinkle of red pepper flakes.

NUTRITION: Calories: 540 Fat: 18g Protein: 27g Sodium: 25mg Total Carbs: 73.5g Dietary Fiber: 6g

8. <u>Quick Quinoa with Cinnamon & Chia</u>

Preparation Time: 15 minutes

Cooking Time: 3 minutes

Servings: 2

INGREDIENTS:

- 2-cups quinoa, pre-cooked
- 1-cup cashew milk
- ½-tsp ground cinnamon
- 1-cup fresh blueberries
- ¼-cup walnuts, toasted
- 2-tsp raw honey
- 1-Tbsp chia seeds

DIRECTIONS:

1. Over medium-low heat, add the quinoa and cashew milk in a saucepan. Stir in the cinnamon, blueberries, and walnuts. Cook slowly for three minutes.
2. Remove the pan from the heat. Stir in the honey. Garnish with chia seeds on top before serving.

NUTRITION: Calories: 887 Fat: 29.5g Protein: 44.Sodium: 85mg Total Carbs: 129.3g Dietary Fiber: 18.5g

9. <u>Plum, Pear & Berry-Baked Brown Rice Recipe</u>

Preparation Time: 12 minutes

Cooking Time: 30 minutes

Servings: 2

INGREDIENTS:

- 1-cup water
- ½-cup brown rice
- A pinch of cinnamon
- ½-tsp pure vanilla extract
- 2-Tbsps pure maple syrup (divided)
- Sliced fruits: berries, pears, or plums
- A bit of salt (optional)

DIRECTIONS:

1. Preheat your oven to 400°F.
2. Bring the water and brown rice mixture to a boil in a pot placed over medium-high heat. Stir in the cinnamon and vanilla extract. Reduce the heat to medium-low. Simmer for 18 minutes, or until the brown rice is tender.
3. Fill two oven-safe bowls with equal portions of the rice. Pour a tablespoon of maple syrup in each bowl. Top the bowls with the sliced fruits and sprinkle over a pinch of salt if you desire.

4. Put the bowls in the oven—Bake for 12 minutes, or until the fruits start caramelizing, and the syrup begins bubbling.

NUTRITION: Calories: 227 Fat: 6.3g Protein: 14.1g Sodium: 80mg Total Carbs: 32.2g Dietary Fiber: 3.6g

10. Swift & Spicy Energy Eggs

Preparation Time: 2 minutes

Cooking Time: 3 minutes

Servings: 1

INGREDIENTS:

- 1-Tbsp milk
- 1-tsp melted butter
- 2-pcs eggs
- A sprinkle of herbs and spices: dried dill, dried oregano, dried parsley, dried thyme, and garlic powder

DIRECTIONS:

1. Preheat your oven to 325°F. Meanwhile, coat the bottom of a baking tray with the milk and butter.
2. Crack the eggs gently over milk and butter coating. Sprinkle the eggs with the dried herbs and garlic powder.
3. Put the tray in the oven. Bake for 3 minutes, or until the eggs cook through.

NUTRITION: Calories: 177 Fat: 5.9g Protein: 8.8g Sodium: 157mg Total Carbs: 22.8g Dietary Fiber: 0.7g

11. Banana Bread Overnight Oats

Preparation Time: 6 hours & 20 minutes

Cooking Time: 0 minutes

Servings: 3

INGREDIENTS:

- ¼-cup plain Greek yogurt
- ¼-tsp flaked sea salt
- 1½-cups nonfat milk
- 1-cup old-fashioned rolled oats
- 1-Tbsp chia seeds
- 2-pcs medium bananas, very ripe and mashed
- 2-Tbsps coconut flakes, unsweetened and toasted
- 2-Tbsps honey
- 2-tsp vanilla extract
- Toppings for serving: roasted pecans, pomegranate seeds, honey, fig halves, and banana slices

DIRECTIONS:

1. Stir in all of the ingredients, excluding the toppings, in a mixing bowl. Mix well until thoroughly combined. Divide the mixture equally between two serving bowls.
2. Cover and refrigerate overnight or for 6 hours.
3. To serve, stir, and put on the toppings.

NUTRITION: Calories: 684 Fat: 22.8g Protein: 34.2g Sodium: 374mg Total Carbs: 99.6g Dietary Fiber: 14.1g

12. Good Grains with Cranberries & Cinnamon

Preparation Time: 8 minutes

Cooking Time: 35 minutes

Servings: 2

INGREDIENTS:

- 1-cup of grains (choice of amaranth, buckwheat, or quinoa)
- 2½-cups coconut water or almond milk
- 1-stick cinnamon

- 2-pcs whole cloves
- 1 star anise pod (optional)
- Fresh fruit: apples, blackberries, cranberries, pears, or persimmons
- Maple syrup (optional)

DIRECTIONS:

1. Bring the grains, coconut water, and the spices to a boil in a saucepan. Cover, then lower the heat to medium-low. Simmer within 25 minutes.
2. To serve, discard the spices and top with fruit slices. If desired, drizzle with the maple syrup.

NUTRITION: Calories: 628 Fat: 20.9g Protein: 31.4g Sodium: 96mg Total Carbs: 112.3g Dietary Fiber: 33.8g

13. **Fresh & Fruity Perky Parfait**

Preparation Time: 20 minutes

Cooking Time: 0 minutes

Servings: 2

INGREDIENTS:

- ½-cup fresh raspberries
- A pinch of cinnamon
- 1-tsp maple syrup
- 2-Tbsps chia seeds
- 16-oz. plain yogurt
- Fresh fruit: sliced blackberries, nectarines, or strawberries

DIRECTIONS:

1. By using a fork, mash the raspberries in a mixing bowl until achieving a jam-like consistency. Add the cinnamon, syrup, and chia seeds. Continue mashing until incorporating all the ingredients. Set aside.

2. In two serving glasses, alternate layers of yogurt and the mixture. Garnish with fresh fruit slices.

NUTRITION: Calories: 315 Fat: 8.7g Protein: 19.6g Sodium: 164mg Total Carbs: 45.8g Dietary Fiber: 6.5g

14. **Seared Syrupy Sage Pork Patties**

Preparation Time: 12 minutes

Cooking Time: 10 minutes

Servings: 4

INGREDIENTS:

- 2-lbs ground pork, pastured
- 3-Tbsps maple syrup, grade B
- 3-Tbsps minced fresh sage
- ¾-tsp sea salt
- ½-tsp garlic powder
- 1-tsp solid cooking fat

DIRECTIONS:

1. Break the ground pork into chunks in a large mixing bowl. Drizzle evenly with the maple syrup. Sprinkle with the spices. Mix well until thoroughly combined. Form the mixture into eight patties. Set aside.
2. Heat the fat in a cast-iron skillet placed over medium heat. Cook the patties for 10 minutes on each side or until browned.

NUTRITION: Calories: 405 Fat: 11.2g Protein: 30.3g Sodium: 240mg Total Carbs: 53.3g Dietary Fiber: 0.8g Net Carbs: 45.5g

15. **Creamy Cinnamon Banana Bowl**

Preparation Time: 5 minutes

Cooking Time: 3 minutes

Servings: 1

INGREDIENTS:

- 1 large banana, ripe
- ¼-tsp cinnamon, ground
- A pinch of Celtic sea salt
- 2-Tbsps coconut butter, melted
- Toppings of your choice: fruit, seed, or nut

DIRECTIONS:

1. Mash the banana in a mixing bowl. Add the cinnamon and Celtic sea salt. Set aside.
2. Heat the coconut butter in a saucepan placed over low heat. Scoop the warm butter to the banana mixture.
3. To serve, top with your favorite fruit, seed, or nut.

NUTRITION: Calories: 564 Fat: 18.8g Protein: 28.2g Sodium: 230mg Total Carbs: 58.2g Dietary Fiber: 15.9g

16. **Turkey with Thyme & Sage Sausage**

Preparation Time: 40 minutes

Cooking Time: 25 minutes

Servings: 4

INGREDIENTS:

- 1-lb ground turkey
- ½-tsp cinnamon
- ½-tsp garlic powder
- 1-tsp fresh rosemary
- 1-tsp fresh thyme
- 1-tsp sea salt
- 2-tsp fresh sage
- 2-Tbsps coconut oil

DIRECTIONS:

1. Stir in all the ingredients, except for the oil, in a mixing bowl. Refrigerate overnight or for 30 minutes.

2. Pour the oil in the mixture. Form the mixture into four patties.
3. In a lightly greased skillet placed over medium heat, cook the patties for 5 minutes on each side, or until their middle portions are no longer pink. You can also cook them by baking in the oven for 25 minutes at 400°F.

NUTRITION: Calories: 284 Fat: 9.4g Protein: 14.2g Sodium: 290mg Total Carbs: 36.9g Dietary Fiber: 0.7g

17. **Spinach Omelet**

Preparation time: 10 minutes

Cooking time: 20 minutes

Servings: 4

INGREDIENTS:

- 8 eggs, whisked
- 1 cup baby spinach
- A pinch of salt and black pepper
- 1 tablespoon olive oil
- 2 spring onions, chopped
- 1 teaspoon sweet paprika
- 1 teaspoon cumin, ground
- 1 tablespoon chives, chopped

DIRECTIONS:

1. Ensure that you heat the pan; add the spring onions, paprika, and cumin, stir and sauté for 5 minutes.
2. Add the eggs, the spinach, salt, and pepper toss spread into the pan, cover it then cook for 15 minutes.
3. Sprinkle the chives on top, divide everything between plates and serve.

NUTRITION: Calories: 345 Fat: 12g Fiber: 1.5g Carbohydrates:8g Protein 13.3g

18. **Pumpkin Pancakes**

Preparation Time: 20 Minutes

Cooking Time: 5 Minutes

Servings: 6

INGREDIENTS:

- 2 ounces hazelnut flour
- 2 ounces flax seeds; ground
- 1-ounce egg white protein
- 1 teaspoon coconut oil
- 1 tablespoon chai masala
- 1 teaspoon vanilla extract
- 1 teaspoon baking powder
- 1 cup coconut cream
- 1 tablespoon swerve
- 1/2 cup pumpkin puree
- 3 eggs
- 5 drops stevia

DIRECTIONS:

1. In a bowl, mix flax seeds with hazelnut flour, egg white protein, baking powder and chai masala and stir.
2. In another bowl, mix coconut cream with vanilla extract, pumpkin puree, eggs, stevia and swerve and stir well.
3. Combine the 2 mixtures and stir well.
4. Heat up a pan with the oil over medium high heat; pour 1/6 of the batter, spread into a circle, cover, reduce heat to low, cook for 3 minutes on each side and transfer to a plate
5. Repeat with the rest of the batter and serve your pumpkin pancakes right away.

NUTRITION: Calories: 400 Cal Fat: 23 g Fiber: 4 g Carbs: 5 g Protein: 21 g

19. Eggs Benedict

Preparation time: 7 minutes

Cooking time: 10 minutes

Servings: 2

INGREDIENTS:

- 2 eggs
- 2 oz bacon, sliced
- 1 tablespoon butter
- ½ teaspoon ground black pepper
- 1 pinch salt
- 1 cup water for cooking

DIRECTIONS:

1. Pour water in the saucepan and add salt. Close the lid and cook it until it starts to boil. Meanwhile, Place sliced bacon in the skillet and roast it for 1 minute over the medium heat from each side. Sprinkle the cooked bacon with the ground black pepper and transfer on the serving plates. Beat the eggs in the boiled water gently to not damage them. Cook the eggs for 3-4 minutes over the medium heat or until the egg white will get white color.
2. Transfer the cooked eggs over the bacon with the help of the ladle.
3. Sprinkle the eggs with the spices if desired.

NUTRITION: Calories:209 Fat: 22g Fiber: 0.8 Carbohydrates: 1.9g Protein: 16.5g

20. Tomato and Eggs Salad

Preparation time: 5 minutes

Cooking time: 0 minutes

Servings: 4

INGREDIENTS:

- 4 eggs, hard-boiled, peeled and cut into wedges
- 2 cups cherry tomatoes, halved
- 1 cup kalamata olives, pitted and halved
- 1 cup baby arugula
- 2 spring onions, chopped
- A pinch of salt and black pepper
- 1 tablespoon avocado oil

DIRECTIONS:

1. In a salad bowl, combine the tomatoes with the eggs and the other ingredients, toss, divide into smaller bowls and serve for breakfast.

NUTRITION: Calories: 126 Fat: 13.3g Fiber: 4.9g Carbohydrates: 10.3g Protein: 6.9g

21. <u>Shallots and Kale Soup</u>

Preparation time: 10 minutes

Cooking time: 20 minutes

Servings: 4

INGREDIENTS:

- 4 cups chicken stock
- 1-pound kale, torn
- 2 shallots, chopped
- A pinch of salt and black pepper
- 1 tablespoon olive oil
- 2 teaspoons coconut amino acids
- 1 tablespoon cilantro, chopped

DIRECTIONS:

1. Heat up a pot with the oil over medium heat; add the shallots and sauté for 5 minutes.
2. Add the kale, stock and the other ingredients bring to a simmer then cook over medium heat for 15 minutes more.
3. Divide the soup into bowls and serve.

NUTRITION: calories 98, fat 4.1, fiber 1.7, carbs 13.1, protein 4.1

22. <u>Mushroom Omelet</u>

Preparation time: 10 minutes

Cooking time: 20 minutes

Servings: 4

INGREDIENTS:

- 2 spring onions, chopped
- ½ pound white mushrooms
- Salt and black pepper to the taste
- 4 eggs, whisked
- 1 tablespoon olive oil
- ½ teaspoon cumin, ground
- 1 tablespoon cilantro, chopped

DIRECTIONS:

1. Ensure that you heat the pan; add the spring onions and the mushrooms, toss and sauté for 5 minutes.
2. Add the eggs and the rest of the ingredients toss gently, spread into the pan, cover it then cook over medium heat for 15 minutes.
3. Slice the omelet, divide it between plates and serve for breakfast.

NUTRITION: Calories 109 Fat 8.1g Fiber 0.8 Carbohydrates 2.9g Protein 7.5g

23. <u>Shrimp and Eggs Mix</u>

Preparation time: 5 minutes

Cooking time: 11 minutes

Servings: 4

INGREDIENTS:

- 8 eggs, whisked
- 1 tablespoon olive oil
- ½ pound shrimp, peeled, deveined and roughly chopped
- ¼ cup green onions, chopped
- 1 teaspoon sweet paprika
- Salt and black pepper to the taste
- 1 tablespoon cilantro, chopped

DIRECTIONS:

1. Ensure that you heat the pan; add the spring onions, toss and sauté for 2 minutes.
2. Add the shrimp, stir then cook for 4 minutes more.
3. Add the eggs, paprika, salt, and pepper, toss then cook for 5 minutes more.
4. Divide the mix between plates, sprinkle the cilantro on top and serve for breakfast.

NUTRITION: Calories: 227 Fat: 13.3g Fiber: 0.4g Carbohydrates: 2.3g Protein: 24.2g

24. <u>Oats with Berries:</u>

Preparation Time: 5 Minutes

Cooking Time: 25 Minutes

Servings: 4

INGREDIENTS:

- 1 cup Steel Cut Oats
- Dash of Salt
- 3 cups Water
- For toppings:
- ½ cup Berries of your choice
- ¼ cup Nuts or Seeds of your choice like Almonds or Hemp Seeds

DIRECTIONS:

1. To begin with, place the oats in a small saucepan and heat it over medium-high heat.
2. Now, toast it for 3 minutes while stirring the pan frequently.
3. Next, pour water to the saucepan and mix well.
4. Allow the mixture to boil. Lower the heat.
5. Allow it to cook for 23 to 25 minutes or until the oats are cooked and tender.
6. Once done cooking, transfer the mixture to the serving bowl and top it with the berries and seeds.
7. Serve it warm or cold.

NUTRITION: Calories: 118Kcal Proteins: 4.1g Carbohydrates: 16.5g Fat: 4.4g

25. **Spiced Morning Chia Pudding**

Preparation Time: 10 Minutes

Cooking Time: 5 Minutes

Servings: 1

INGREDIENTS:

- ½ tsp. Cinnamon
- 1 ½ cups Cashew Milk
- 1/8 tsp. Cardamom, grounded
- 1/3 cup Chia Seeds
- 1/8 tsp. Cloves, grounded
- 2 tbsp. Maple Syrup

- 1 tsp. Turmeric

DIRECTIONS:

1. To begin with, combine all the ingredients in a medium bowl until well mixed.
2. Next, spoon the mixture into a container and allow it to sit overnight.
3. In the morning, transfer to a cup and serve with toppings of your choice.

Tip: You can top it with toppings of your choice like coconut flakes or seeds etc.

NUTRITION: Calories: 237Kcal Proteins: 8.1g Carbohydrates: 28.9g Fat: 8.1g

26. **Quick Burrito**

Preparation Time:10 Minutes

Cooking Time: 11 Minutes

Servings: 1

INGREDIENTS:

- 1/4-pound beef meat; ground
- 1 teaspoon sweet paprika
- 1 teaspoon cumin; ground
- 1 teaspoon onion powder
- 1 small red onion; julienned
- 3 eggs
- 1 teaspoon coconut oil
- 1 teaspoon garlic powder
- 1 teaspoon cilantro; chopped.
- Salt and black pepper to the taste.

DIRECTIONS:

1. Heat up a pan over medium heat; add beef and brown for a few minutes
2. Add salt, pepper, cumin, garlic and onion powder and paprika; stir, cook for 4 minutes more and take off heat.
3. In a bowl, mix eggs with salt and pepper and whisk well.
4. Heat up a pan with the oil over medium heat; add egg, spread evenly and cook for 6 minutes

5. Transfer your egg burrito to a plate, divide beef mix, add onion and cilantro, roll and serve

NUTRITION: Calories: 280 Cal Fat: 12 g Fiber: 4 Carbs: 7 g Protein: 14 g

27. <u>Blueberry and Cashew Mix</u>

Preparation time: 10 minutes

Cooking time: 12 minutes

Servings: 2

INGREDIENTS:

- 2 bananas, peeled and sliced
- ¼ cup cashews
- ¼ cup blueberries
- 1 tablespoon almond butter
- 1/3 cup coconut flakes, unsweetened
- 1 cup coconut milk, unsweetened

DIRECTIONS:

1. In a small pot, mix the berries with the coconut flakes, milk, cashews, almond butter and bananas. Mix together and bring to a simmer over medium heat. Cook for 12 minutes, divide into bowls and serve for breakfast.
2. Enjoy!

NUTRITION: Calories: 370 Cal Fat: 23 g Fiber: 6 g Carbs: 40 g Protein: 8 g

28. <u>Oatmeal Pancakes</u>

Preparation Time: 5 Minutes

Cooking Time: 25 Minutes

Servings: 2

INGREDIENTS:

- 1 ½ cups Rolled Oats, whole-grain
- 2 Eggs, large & pastured
- 2 tsp. Baking Powder
- 1 Banana, ripe
- 2 tbsp. Water

- ¼ cup Maple Syrup
- 1 tsp. Vanilla Extract
- 2 tbsp. Extra Virgin Olive Oil

DIRECTIONS:

1. To make this delicious breakfast dish, you need to first blend all the ingredients in a high-speed blender for a minute or two or until you get a smooth batter. Tip: To blend easily, pour egg, banana, and all other liquid ingredients first and finally add oats at the end.
2. Now, take a large skillet and heat it over medium-low heat.
3. Once the skillet is hot, ¼ cup of the batter into it and cook it for 3 to 4 minutes per side or until bubbles start appearing in the middle portion.
4. Turn the pancake and cook the other side also.
5. Serve warm.

NUTRITION: Calories: 201Kcal Proteins: 5g Carbohydrates: 28g Fat: 8g

29. <u>No Cook Overnight Oats</u>

Preparation Time: 5 Minutes

Cooking Time: 0 Minute

Servings: 1

INGREDIENTS:

- 1 ½ c. low fat milk
- 5 whole almond pieces
- 1 tsp. chia seeds
- 2 tbsps. Oats
- 1 tsp. sunflower seeds
- 1 tbsp. raisins

DIRECTIONS:

1. In a jar or mason bottle with cap, mix all ingredients.
2. Refrigerate overnight.
3. Enjoy for breakfast. Will keep in the fridge for up to 3 days.

NUTRITION: Calories: 271 Cal Fat: 9.8 g Carbohydrates:35.4 g Protein:16.7 g Sugars:9 g

30. Grilled Veggie Skewers

Preparation Time: 10 minutes

Cooking Time: 15 minutes

Servings: 5

INGREDIENTS:

For Marinade Mixture:

- 3 garlic cloves, chopped
- 1 (1-inchpieces fresh ginger, chopped
- 1 teaspoon ground cumin
- 1 teaspoon ground coriander
- 1teaspoon sweet paprika
- 1/8 teaspoon red chili powder
- Salt and freshly ground black pepper, to taste
- ¼ cup fresh lemon juice
- ¼ cup organic olive oil
- ½ lot of fresh cilantro
- ½ couple of fresh parsley

For Vegetables:

- 2 medium red bell pepper, seeded and cut into 1-inch pieces
- 2 medium zucchinis, cut into 1/3-inch thick round slices
- 1-pound small mushrooms
- 1 large yellow onion, sliced into 1-inch pieces
- 1 large eggplant, quartered lengthwise and cut into ½-inch thick slices diagonally

DIRECTIONS:

1. For marinade mixture in the blender, add all ingredients except herbs and pulse till well combined.
2. Add fresh herbs and pulse till smooth.
3. In a sizable bowl, add vegetables and marinade and toss to coat well.

4. Refrigerate, covered approximately 4 hours.
5. Preheat the grill to medium-low heat. Grease the grill grate.
6. Thread the skewers for around 15 minutes, flipping occasionally.

NUTRITION: Calories: 254 Fat: 5g Carbohydrates: 25g Fiber: 6g Protein: 27g

31. Spiced Popcorn

Preparation Time: 5 minutes

Cooking Time: 2 minutes

Servings: 2-3

INGREDIENTS:

- 3 tablespoons coconut oil
- ½ cup popping corn
- 1 tbsp. olive oil
- 1 teaspoon ground turmeric
- ¼ teaspoon garlic powder
- Salt, to taste

DIRECTIONS:

1. In a pan, melt coconut oil on medium-high heat.
2. Add popping corn and cover the pan tightly.
3. Cook, shaking the pan occasionally for around 1-2 minutes or till corn kernels begin to pop.
4. Remove from heat and transfer right into a large heatproof bowl.
5. Add essential olive oil and spices and mix well.
6. Serve immediately

NUTRITION: Calories: 200 Fat: 4g Carbohydrates: 12g Fiber: 1g Protein: 6g

32. Early Morning Pesto Eggs

Preparation Time: 5 minutes

Cooking Time: 5 minutes

Servings: 2

INGREDIENTS:

- 2 large whole eggs
- 1/2 tablespoon almond butter
- 1/2 tablespoon pesto
- 1 tablespoon creamed coconut almond milk
- Sunflower seeds and pepper as needed

DIRECTIONS:

1. Take a bowl and crack open your egg.
2. Season with a pinch of sunflower seeds and pepper.
3. Pour eggs into a pan.
4. Add almond butter and introduce heat.
5. Cook on low heat and gently add pesto.
6. Once the egg is cooked and scrambled, remove heat.
7. Spoon in coconut cream and mix well.
8. Turn on the heat and cook on LOW for a while until you have a creamy texture.
9. Serve and enjoy!

NUTRITION: Calories: 467 Cal Fat: 41 g Carbohydrates: 3 g Protein: 20 g

33. **Grilled Eggplant Caprese**

Preparation Time: 10 Minutes

Cooking Time: 10 Minutes

Servings: 4

INGREDIENTS:

- 1 eggplant aubergine, small/medium
- 1 tomato large
- 2 basil leaves or a little more as needed
- 4-oz mozzarella
- good quality olive oil
- Pepper and salt to taste

DIRECTIONS:

1. Cut the ends of the eggplant and then cut it lengthwise into ¼-inch thick slices. Discard the smaller pieces that's mostly skin and short.

2. Slice the tomatoes and mozzarella into thin slices just like the eggplant.
3. On medium-high the fire, place a griddle and let it heat up.
4. Brush eggplant slices with olive oil and place on grill. Grill for 3 minutes. Turnover and grill for a minute. Add a slice of cheese on one side and tomato on the other side. Continue cooking for another 2 minutes.
5. Sprinkle with basil leaves. Season with pepper and salt.
6. Fold eggplant in half and skewer with a cocktail stick.
7. Serve and enjoy.

NUTRITION: Calories: 82 Fat: 0g Carbohydrates: 11g Protein: 11g Sugar: 7g Fiber 5g

34. **Hot Kale Pan**

Preparation time: 5 minutes

Cooking time: 23 minutes

Servings: 4

INGREDIENTS:

- 1 red onion, chopped
- 1-pound kale, roughly torn
- 1 cup baby bella mushrooms, halved
- A pinch of salt and black pepper
- 1 tablespoon olive oil
- 3 garlic cloves, minced
- ½ teaspoon hot paprika
- ½ tablespoon red pepper flakes, crushed
- 1 tablespoon dill, chopped
- 3 tablespoons coconut amino acids

DIRECTIONS:

1. Ensure that you heat the pan; add the onion and the garlic and sauté for 5 minutes.
2. Add the mushrooms and sauté them for 3 minutes more.
3. Add the kale and the other ingredients, toss, cook over medium heat for 15 minutes more, divide into bowls and serve.

NUTRITION: Calories: 100 Fat: 3g Fiber: 1g Carbohydrates: 2g Protein: 6

35. Egg Porridge

Preparation Time: 14 minutes

Cooking Time: 0 Minute

Servings: 2

INGREDIENTS:

- 2 eggs
- 2 tablespoons ghee; melted
- 1/3 cup heavy cream
- 1 tablespoon stevia
- A pinch of cinnamon; ground

DIRECTIONS:

1. In a bowl, mix eggs with stevia and heavy cream and whisk well.
2. Heat up a pan with the ghee over medium high heat; add egg mix and cook until they are done
3. Transfer to 2 bowls, sprinkle cinnamon on top and serve

NUTRITION: Calories: 340 Cal Fat: 12 g Fiber: 10; Carbohydrates: 3 g Protein: 14 g

LUNCH RECIPES

36. Kale Soup

Preparation time: 10 minutes

Cooking time: 15 minutes

Servings: 4

INGREDIENTS:

- 1 pound kale, chopped
- Salt and black pepper to the taste
- 5 cups vegetable stock
- 2 carrots, sliced
- 1 yellow onion, chopped
- 1 tablespoon olive oil
- 1 tablespoon parsley, chopped
- 1 tablespoon lemon juice

DIRECTIONS:

1. Heat up a pot with the oil over medium heat, add the carrots and the onion, stir and sauté for 5 minutes.
2. Add the kale and the other ingredients, toss, bring to a simmer and cook over medium heat for 10 minutes more.
3. Ladle the soup into bowls and serve.

NUTRITION: calories 210, fat 7, fiber 2, carbs 10, protein 8

37. Salmon with Balsamic Fennel

Preparation time: 10 minutes

Cooking time: 20 minutes

Servings: 4

INGREDIENTS:

- 4 salmon fillets, boneless
- 1 tablespoon olive oil
- 2 fennel bulbs, shredded
- 1 tablespoon balsamic vinegar
- 1 tablespoon lime juice
- ½ teaspoon cumin, ground
- ½ teaspoon oregano, dried
- 1 tablespoon chives, chopped
- Salt and black pepper to the taste

DIRECTIONS:

1. Heat up a pan with the oil over medium heat, add the fennel, stir and sauté for 5 minutes.
2. Add the fish and sear it for 2 minutes on each side.
3. Add the remaining ingredients, cook everything for 10 minutes more, divide between plates and serve.

NUTRITION: calories 200, fat 2, fiber 4, carbs 10, protein 8

38. Carrot Soup

Preparation time: 10 minutes

Cooking time: 25 minutes

Servings: 4

INGREDIENTS:

- 1 pound carrots, peeled and sliced
- 2 tablespoons olive oil
- 1 yellow onion, chopped
- 1 teaspoon rosemary, dried
- 1 teaspoon cumin, ground
- 2 garlic cloves, minced
- A pinch of salt and black pepper
- 5 cups vegetable stock
- ½ teaspoon turmeric powder
- 1 cup coconut milk
- 1 tablespoon chives, chopped

DIRECTIONS:

1. Heat up a pot with the oil over medium heat, add the onion and the garlic and sauté for 5 minutes.
2. Add the carrots, the stock and the other ingredients except the chives, stir, bring to

a simmer and cook over medium heat for 20 minutes more.

3. Divide the soup into bowls, sprinkle the chives on top and serve for lunch.

NUTRITION: calories 210, fat 8, fiber 6, carbs 10, protein 7

39. Leeks Cream Soup

Preparation time: 10 minutes

Cooking time: 20 minutes

Servings: 4

INGREDIENTS:

- 4 leeks, sliced
- 1 yellow onion, chopped
- 1 tablespoon avocado oil
- A pinch of salt and black pepper
- 2 garlic cloves, minced
- 4 cups vegetable soup
- ½ cup coconut milk
- ½ teaspoon nutmeg, ground
- ¼ teaspoon red pepper, crushed
- ½ teaspoon rosemary, dried
- 1 tablespoon parsley, chopped

DIRECTIONS:

1. Heat up a pot with the oil over medium-high heat, add the onion and the garlic and sauté for 2 minutes.
2. Add the leeks, stir and sauté for 3 minutes more.
3. Add the stock and the rest of the ingredients except the parsley, bring to a simmer and cook over medium heat for 15 minutes more.
4. Blend the soup with an immersion blender, divide the soup into bowls, sprinkle the parsley on top and serve.

NUTRITION: calories 268, fat 11.8, fiber 4.5, carbs 37.4, protein 6.1

40. Turkey and Artichokes

Preparation time: 10 minutes

Cooking time: 40 minutes

Servings: 4

INGREDIENTS:

- 1 yellow onion, sliced
- 1 pound turkey breast, skinless, boneless and roughly cubed
- 2 tablespoons olive oil
- Salt and black pepper to the taste
- 1 cup canned artichoke hearts, drained and halved
- ½ teaspoon nutmeg, ground
- ½ teaspoon sweet paprika
- 1 teaspoon cumin, ground
- 1 tablespoon cilantro, chopped

DIRECTIONS:

1. In a roasting pan, combine the turkey with the onion, artichokes and the other ingredients, toss and at 350 degrees F for 40 minutes.
2. Divide everything between plates and serve.

NUTRITION: calories 345, fat 12, fiber 3, carbs 12, protein 14

41. Smoked Salmon Salad

Preparation time: 10 minutes

Cooking time: 0 minutes

Servings: 4

INGREDIENTS:

- 2 cups smoked salmon, skinless, boneless and cut into strips
- 1 yellow onion, chopped
- 1 avocado, peeled, pitted and cubed
- 1 cup cherry tomatoes, halved
- 1 tablespoon olive oil
- 2 cups baby spinach
- A pinch of salt and cayenne pepper

- 1 tablespoon balsamic vinegar

DIRECTIONS:

1. In a salad bowl, mix the salmon with the onion, the avocado and the other ingredients, toss, divide between plates and serve for lunch.

NUTRITION: calories 260, fat 2, fiber 8, carbs 17, protein 11

42. **Shrimp with Zucchini**

Preparation time: 10 minutes

Cooking time: 17 minutes

Servings: 4

INGREDIENTS:

- 1 pound shrimp, peeled and deveined
- 1 tablespoon lemon juice
- 2 zucchinis, sliced
- 1 yellow onion, roughly chopped
- 1 tablespoon olive oil
- 1 teaspoon turmeric powder
- A pinch of salt and black pepper
- 1 tablespoons capers, drained
- 2 tablespoons pine nuts

DIRECTIONS:

1. Heat up a pan with the oil over medium-high heat, add the onion and the zucchini, stir and sauté for 5 minutes.
2. Add the shrimp and the other ingredients, toss, cook everything for 12 minutes more, divide into bowls and serve for lunch.

NUTRITION: calories 162, fat 3, fiber 4, carbs 12, protein 7

43. **Turmeric Broccoli and Leeks Stew**

Preparation time: 10 minutes

Cooking time: 25 minutes

Servings: 4

INGREDIENTS:

- 1 tablespoon olive oil
- 1 pound broccoli florets
- ½ teaspoon coriander, ground
- 1 yellow onion, chopped
- 2 leeks, sliced
- 4 garlic cloves, minced
- ½ teaspoon turmeric powder
- A pinch of cayenne pepper
- 1 cup tomato passata
- A pinch of salt and black pepper
- 1 tablespoon lemon juice
- 1 tablespoon cilantro, chopped

DIRECTIONS:

1. Heat up a pot with the oil over medium heat, add the onion, garlic, leeks and the turmeric and sauté for 5 minutes.
2. Add the broccoli and the other ingredients, toss, bring to a simmer and cook over medium heat for 25 minutes more.
3. Divide into bowls and serve for lunch.

NUTRITION: calories 113, fat 4.1, fiber 4.5, carbs 17.7, protein 4.4

44. **Salmon and Green Beans**

Preparation time: 10 minutes

Cooking time: 26 minutes

Servings: 4

INGREDIENTS:

- 2 tablespoons olive oil
- 1 yellow onion, chopped
- 4 salmon fillets, boneless
- 1 cup green beans, trimmed and halved
- 2 garlic cloves, minced
- ½ cup chicken stock
- 1 teaspoon chili powder
- 1 teaspoon sweet paprika
- A pinch of salt and black pepper
- 1 tablespoon cilantro, chopped

DIRECTIONS:

1. Heat up a pan with the oil over medium heat, add onion, stir and sauté for 2 minutes.
2. Add the fish and sear it for 2 minutes on each side.
3. Add the rest of the ingredients, toss gently and bake everything at 360 degrees F for 20 minutes.
4. Divide everything between plates and serve for lunch.

NUTRITION: calories 322, fat 18.3, fiber 2, carbs 5.8, protein 35.7

45. Chicken Stew

Preparation time: 10 minutes

Cooking time: 45 minutes

Servings: 4

INGREDIENTS:

- 1 tablespoon olive oil
- 1 pound chicken thighs, skinless, boneless and cubed
- 2 garlic cloves, minced
- 1 small yellow onion, chopped
- 1 green bell pepper, chopped
- 1 red bell pepper, chopped
- ½ teaspoon cumin, ground
- ½ teaspoon sweet paprika
- 2 cups chicken stock
- A pinch of salt and black pepper
- 1 tablespoon lemon juice
- 1 cup coconut milk
- 1 tablespoon cilantro, chopped

DIRECTIONS:

1. Heat up a pot with the oil over medium heat, add the onion, garlic and the meat and brown for 10 minutes stirring often.
2. Add the rest of the ingredients except the coconut milk and the cilantro, stir, bring to a simmer and cook over medium for 30 minutes more.

3. Add the coconut milk and the cilantro, stir, simmer the stew for 5 minutes more, divide into bowls and serve for lunch.

NUTRITION: calories 419, fat 26.8, fiber 2.7, carbs 10.7, protein 35.5

46. Spiced Turkey Stew

Preparation time: 10 minutes

Cooking time: 45 minutes

Servings: 6

INGREDIENTS:

- 1 pound turkey breast, skinless, boneless and cubed
- 1 yellow onion, chopped
- 2 tablespoons olive oil
- ½ teaspoon mustard seeds
- 1 teaspoon ginger, grated
- 2 garlic cloves, minced
- 1 green chili pepper, chopped
- 1 teaspoon sweet paprika
- 1 teaspoon coriander, ground
- ½ teaspoon cardamom, ground
- ½ teaspoon turmeric powder
- A pinch of salt and black pepper
- 1 teaspoon lemon juice
- 1 cup chicken stock
- 1 tablespoon parsley, chopped

DIRECTIONS:

1. Heat up a pot with the oil over medium-high heat, add the onion, the meat, mustard seeds, ginger, garlic, paprika, coriander, cardamom and the turmeric, stir and brown for 10 minutes.
2. Add all the other ingredients, toss, simmer over medium heat for 35 minutes more, divide into bowls and serve.

NUTRITION: calories 202, fat 9.4, fiber 1.7, carbs 9.3, protein 20.3

47. Beans and Salmon Pan

Preparation time: 10 minutes

Cooking time: 25 minutes

Servings: 4

INGREDIENTS:

- 1 cup canned black beans, drained and rinsed
- 4 garlic cloves, minced
- 1 yellow onion, chopped
- 2 tablespoons olive oil
- 4 salmon fillets, boneless
- ½ teaspoon coriander, ground
- 1 teaspoon turmeric powder
- 2 tomatoes, cubed
- ½ cup chicken stock
- A pinch of salt and black pepper
- ½ teaspoon cumin seeds
- 1 tablespoon chives, chopped

DIRECTIONS:

1. Heat up a pan with the oil over medium heat, add the onion and the garlic and sauté for 5 minutes.
2. Add the fish and sear it for 2 minutes on each side.
3. Add the beans and the other ingredients, toss gently and cook for 10 minutes more.
4. Divide the mix between plates and serve right away for lunch.

NUTRITION: calories 219, fat 8, fiber 8, carbs 12, protein 8

48. **Turmeric Cauliflower and Cod Stew**

Preparation time: 5 minutes

Cooking time: 30 minutes

Servings: 4

INGREDIENTS:

- ½ pound cauliflower florets
- 1 pound cod fillets, boneless, skinless and cubed

- 1 tablespoons olive oil
- 1 yellow onion, chopped
- ½ teaspoon cumin seeds
- 1 green chili, chopped
- ¼ teaspoon turmeric powder
- 2 tomatoes chopped
- A pinch of salt and black pepper
- ½ cup chicken stock
- 1 tablespoon cilantro, chopped

DIRECTIONS:

1. Heat up a pot with the oil over medium heat, add the onion, chili, cumin and turmeric, stir and cook for 5 minutes.
2. Add the cauliflower, the fish and the other ingredients, toss, bring to a simmer and cook over medium heat for 25 minutes more.
3. Divide the stew into bowls and serve.

NUTRITION: calories 281, fat 6, fiber 4, carbs 8, protein 12

49. **Chicken Chili**

Preparation time: 10 minutes

Cooking time: 1 hour

Servings: 6

INGREDIENTS:

- 1 yellow onion, chopped
- 2 tablespoons olive oil
- 2 garlic cloves, minced
- 1 pound chicken breast, skinless, boneless and cubed
- 1 green bell pepper, chopped
- 2 cups chicken stock
- 1 tablespoon cocoa powder
- 2 tablespoons chili powder
- 1 teaspoon smoked paprika
- 1 cup canned tomatoes, chopped
- 1 tablespoon cilantro, chopped
- A pinch of salt and black pepper

DIRECTIONS:

1. Heat up a pot with the oil over medium heat, add the onion and the garlic and sauté for 5 minutes.
2. Add the meat and brown it for 5 minutes more.
3. Add the rest of the ingredients, toss, cook over medium heat for 40 minutes.
4. Divide the chili into bowls and serve for lunch.

NUTRITION: calories 300, fat 2, fiber 10, carbs 15, protein 11

50. Green Beans Soup

Preparation time: 10 minutes

Cooking time: 35 minutes

Servings: 6

INGREDIENTS:

- 1 yellow onion, chopped
- 1-pound green beans, trimmed and halved
- 1 carrot, peeled and grated
- 2 tomatoes, cubed
- 1 tablespoon olive oil
- 2 teaspoons cumin, ground
- 6 cups veggie stock
- ¼ teaspoon chipotle chili powder
- 1 tablespoon cilantro, chopped

DIRECTIONS:

1. Heat up a pot with the oil over medium heat, add the onion and the carrot and sauté for 5 minutes.
2. Add the green beans and the rest of the ingredients, toss, bring to a simmer and cook over medium heat for 30 minutes.
3. Ladle the soup into bowls and serve.

NUTRITION: calories 224, fat 2, fiber 12, carbs 10, protein 17

51. Grilled Avocado Sandwich

Preparation Time: 10 minutes

Cooking Time: 15 minutes

Servings: 4

INGREDIENTS:

- 8 slices of pumpernickel bread
- 1 cup sauerkraut, drained & rinsed
- 1 cup hummus
- 1 teaspoon dairy-free margarine
- 1 avocado, peeled & sliced into 16 pieces

DIRECTIONS:

1. Preheat your oven to 450 degrees F.
2. Apply margarine on one side of your bread slices.
3. Keep 4 slices on your baking sheet. The margarine side should be down.
4. Distribute half of the hummus over the bread slices.
5. Place sauerkraut on the hummus.
6. Keep avocado slices over your sauerkraut.
7. Spread hummus on the remaining slices.
8. Keep the hummus side down on your slices of avocado.
9. Bake for 7 minutes.
10. Flip over and bake for another 6 minutes.

NUTRITION: Calories 340 Carbohydrates 39g Total Fat 16g Protein 10g Fiber 11g Sugar 1g Sodium 781mg Potassium 552mg

52. Cauliflower Steaks with Tamarind and Beans

Preparation Time: 5 minutes

Cooking Time: 25 minutes

Servings: 2

INGREDIENTS:

- ½ cup of olive oil
- 1/5 lb. cauliflower head
- 1 teaspoon black pepper, ground
- 2 teaspoons of kosher salt
- 3 cloves of garlic, chopped

- ½ lb. green beans, trimmed
- 1/3 cup parsley, chopped
- ¾ teaspoon lemon zest, grated
- 1/5 lb. parmesan, grated
- ¼ lb. panko breadcrumbs
- 1/3 cup tamarind
- 1 lb. white beans, rinsed & drained
- 1 teaspoon of Dijon mustard
- 2 tablespoons of margarine

DIRECTIONS:

1. Preheat your oven to 425 degrees F.
2. Take out the leaves and trim the stem ends of your cauliflower.
3. Keep the core side down on your working surface.
4. Slice from the center top to down with a knife.
5. Keep it on a baking sheet.
6. Apply 1 tablespoon oil on both sides. Season with pepper and salt.
7. Roast for 25 minutes. Turn halfway through.
8. Toss the green beans in the meantime with 1 tablespoon of oil and pepper.
9. Keep on your baking sheet in a single layer.
10. Whisk the lemon zest, garlic, parsley, salt, pepper, and oil together in a bowl.
11. Keep half of this mix in another bowl.
12. Add Parmesan and panko to the first bowl. Use your hands to mix.
13. Add tamarind and white beans to the second bowl. Coat well by tossing.
14. Now whisk together the mustard and margarine.
15. Spread your margarine mix over the cauliflower.
16. Sprinkle the panko mix over the cauliflower.
17. Add the white bean mix to the sheet with beans. Combine.
18. Keep sheet in the oven and roast for 5 minutes.
19. Divide the beans, cauliflower, and tamarind among plates.

NUTRITION: Calories 1366 Carbohydrates 166g Cholesterol 6mg Total Fat 67g Protein 59g Fiber 41g Sugar 20g Sodium 2561mg

53. **Smoked Salmon Tartine**

Preparation Time: 5 minutes

Cooking Time: 20 minutes

Servings: 2

INGREDIENTS:

- 1/3 pumpkin
- 2 tablespoons of dairy-free margarine
- 1-1/2 tablespoons chives, minced
- ¼ lb. cashew paste
- Thinly sliced smoked salmon
- ½ clove of garlic, minced
- ½ lemon zest
- 2 tablespoons red onion, chopped
- 2 tablespoons capers, drained
- ½ boiled egg, chopped
- Black pepper and kosher salt

DIRECTIONS:

1. Bring together the lemon zest, garlic and cashew paste in a bowl.
2. Season with pepper and salt. Stir in the chives gently and set aside.
3. Now season the boiled egg and red onion with salt.
4. Grate your pumpkin.
5. Squeeze the pumpkin and remove any excess liquid. Season with pepper and salt.
6. Heat the margarine over medium temperature.
7. Add the pumpkin. Use a spatula to shape roughly into a circle.
8. Use the backside of a spoon to press on your mixture.
9. Cook covered for 10 minutes.

10. Flip and cook for another 8 minutes. It should be crispy and golden brown.
11. Take out and let it cool.
12. Spread the paste mix on top.
13. Layer your smoked salmon over this.
14. Sprinkle with capers, the boiled egg, and red onion.
15. Garnish with chives.
16. Cut into small wedges before serving.

NUTRITION: Calories 734 Carbohydrates 37g Cholesterol 115mg Total Fat 54g Protein 25g Sugar 3g Fiber 5g Sodium 1641mg

54. <u>Healthy Chicken Marsala</u>

Preparation Time: 5 minutes

Cooking Time: 25 minutes

Servings: 4

INGREDIENTS:

- 1-1/2 chicken breasts, boneless & skinless
- 2 tablespoons of dairy-free margarine
- ½ lb. shiitake mushrooms, sliced & stemmed
- 1 lb. baby Bella mushrooms, sliced & stemmed
- 2 tablespoons of extra virgin olive oil
- 3 cloves of garlic, chopped
- 1 cup shallot, chopped
- 2 cups of chicken broth, low-sodium
- ¾ cup dry marsala wine
- Black pepper, kosher salt, chopped parsley leaves

DIRECTIONS:

1. Dry your chicken breasts using a paper towel.
2. Slice them horizontally into half.
3. Keep each piece between parchment paper. Use your meat mallet to pound until you have ¼ inch thickness.
4. Season all sides with black pepper and kosher salt.

5. Dredge in some whole wheat flour. Keep aside.
6. Heat your skillet over medium temperature.
7. Pour olive oil and margarine in your pan.
8. Sauté the chicken for 5 minutes. Work in batches, not overcrowding your pan.
9. Transfer to a baking sheet. Set aside.
10. Wipe off excess cooking fat from your pan. Bring back to heat.
11. Add the remaining margarine and the mushrooms.
12. Sauté over high temperature. Season with black pepper and salt.
13. Add the garlic and chopped shallot to your pan.
14. Sauté 3 minutes. Include the marsala wine. Bring down the heat for a minute.
15. Include the chicken broth and cook for 5 minutes.
16. Transfer chicken cutlets to the pan. Spoon over the sauce.
17. Garnish with parsley.

NUTRITION: Calories 546 Carbohydrates 41g Cholesterol 31mg Total Fat 38g Protein 10g Sugar 6g Fiber 5g Sodium 535mg

55. <u>Grilled Salmon Burgers</u>

Preparation Time: 10 minutes

Cooking Time: 10 minutes

Servings: 4

INGREDIENTS:

- 1 lb. salmon fillet, skinless and cubed
- 1 tablespoon Dijon mustard
- 1 tablespoon lime peel, grated
- 1 tablespoon ginger, peeled & minced
- 1 tablespoon cilantro, chopped
- 1 teaspoon soy sauce, low-sodium
- ½ teaspoon coriander, ground
- Cilantro leaves and lime wedges
- Pepper and salt to taste

DIRECTIONS:

1. Preheat your barbecue grill on medium heat.
2. Apply cooking spray on the grill's rack lightly.
3. Pulse the salmon in your food processor. It should grind coarsely.
4. Take out the salmon and keep in a bowl.
5. Mix in the lime peel, mustard, cilantro, ginger, coriander, and soy sauce.
6. Create 4 patties.
7. Season with pepper and salt.
8. Grill your burgers, turning once on medium heat. 4 minutes for each side.
9. Garnish with cilantro leaves and lime wedges.

NUTRITION: Calories: 395 Cholesterol: 60 mg Carbohydrates: 1 g Fat: 7 g Sugar: 0 g Fiber: 0 g Protein: 23 g

56. Tuna Steaks

Preparation Time: 15 minutes

Cooking Time: 15 minutes

Servings: 2

INGREDIENTS:

- 1-1/2 cups water
- 1 tablespoon lemon juice
- Pepper and salt to taste
- 1 teaspoon cayenne pepper
- 2 tuna steaks
- 3 kumquats, seeded, sliced, rinsed
- 1/3 cup cilantro, chopped

DIRECTIONS:

1. Mix lemon juice, cayenne pepper and water over medium heat in a saucepan.
2. Season with pepper and salt. Boil.
3. Now include the tuna steaks into this mix.
4. Sprinkle cilantro and kumquats.
5. Cook for 15 minutes. The fish should flake easily with your fork.

NUTRITION: Calories: 141 Cholesterol: 50 mg Carbohydrates: 6 g Fat: 1 g Sugar: 3 g Fiber: 2 g Protein: 27 g

57. Air Fryer Salmon

Preparation Time: 6 minutes

Cooking Time: 5 minutes

Servings: 2

INGREDIENTS:

- 1/3 lb. filets of salmon
- ¼ cup of margarine
- ¼ cup of pistachios, chopped finely
- 1-1/2 tablespoons of minced dill
- 2 tablespoons of lemon juice

DIRECTIONS:

1. Preheat your air fryer to 400 degrees F.
2. Spray olive oil on the basket.
3. Season your salmon with pepper to taste. You can also apply the all-purpose seasoning.
4. Combine the margarine, lemon juice, and dill in a bowl.
5. Pour a spoonful on the fillets.
6. Top the fillets with chopped pistachios. Be generous.
7. Spray olive oil on the salmon lightly.
8. Air fry your fillets now for 5 minutes.
9. Take out the salmon carefully with a spatula from your air fryer.
10. Keep on a plate. Garnish with dill.

NUTRITION: Calories 305 Carbohydrates 1g Cholesterol 43mg Total Fat 21g Protein 28g Fiber 2g Sugar 3g Sodium 92mg

58. Rosemary Garlic Lamb Chops

Preparation Time: 3 minutes

Cooking Time: 10 minutes

Servings: 2

INGREDIENTS:

- 4 chops of lamb
- 1 teaspoon olive oil
- 2 teaspoon garlic puree
- Fresh garlic
- Fresh rosemary

DIRECTIONS:

1. Keep your lamb chops in the fryer grill pan.
2. Season the chops with pepper and salt. Brush some olive oil.
3. Add some garlic puree on each chop.
4. Cover the grill pan gaps with garlic cloves and rosemary sprigs.
5. Refrigerate to marinate.
6. Take out after 1 hour. Keep in the fryer and cook for 5 minutes.
7. Use your spatula to turn the chops over.
8. Add some olive oil and cook for another 5 minutes.
9. Set aside for a minute.
10. Take out the rosemary and garlic before serving.

NUTRITION: Calories 678 Carbohydrates 1g Cholesterol 257mg Total Fat 38g Protein 83g Sugar 0g Sodium 200mg

59. **Mushroom Farro Risotto**

Preparation Time: 2 minutes

Cooking Time: 28 minutes

Servings: 5

INGREDIENTS:

- 3 tablespoons of melted coconut oil
- 4 cups chicken broth, low sodium
- ¾ lb. baby Bella mushrooms, trimmed & sliced
- ½ yellow onion, chopped
- 3 cloves of garlic, chopped
- 1 tablespoon thyme, chopped

- ¾ cup of dry white wine
- 1-1/2 cups organic farro
- 1 teaspoon lemon juice
- ¾ cup vegan parmesan
- ¾ cup peas
- Ground black pepper, kosher salt, chopped parsley

DIRECTIONS:

1. Keep your chicken broth in a saucepan. Simmer over low heat.
2. Heat the coconut oil over medium temperature in a pot.
3. Add kosher salt and onion. Sauté for 6 minutes. Stir often.
4. Bring up the heat to high. Now add the mushrooms. Combine by stirring.
5. Cook for another 2 minutes. The mushrooms should become soft.
6. Add the thyme and garlic. Sauté for a minute, stirring occasionally.
7. Include the toast and farro and cook for 1 more minute. Keep stirring.
8. Pour in the white wine. Cook for 3 minutes. Stir often. The wine needs to be absorbed completely.
9. Add the hot broth to your pot. Combine well.
10. Bring down the heat and cook for 30 minutes. Stir every 15 minutes.
11. Add the lemon juice and grated parmesan. Stir to combine.
12. Fold in the peas. Season with pepper and salt.
13. Take out the pot from heat. Let it sit covered for 5 minutes.
14. Garnish with thyme leaves and parsley.

NUTRITION: Calories 397 Carbohydrates 29g Cholesterol 32mg Total Fat 25g Protein 14g Sugar 5g Fiber 5g Sodium 429mg

DINNER RECIPES

60. Crispy Cheese-Crusted Fish Fillet

Preparation Time: 5-minutes

Cooking Time: 10-minutes

Servings: 4

INGREDIENTS:

- ¼-cup whole-wheat breadcrumbs
- ¼-cup Parmesan cheese, grated
- ¼-tsp sea salt
- ¼-tsp ground pepper
- 1-Tbsp olive oil
- 4-pcs tilapia fillets

DIRECTIONS:

1. Preheat the oven to 375°F.
2. Stir in the breadcrumbs, Parmesan cheese, salt, pepper, and olive oil in a mixing bowl. Mix well until blended thoroughly.
3. Coat the fillets with the mixture, and lay each on a lightly sprayed baking sheet. Place the sheet in the oven. Bake for 10 minutes until the fillets cook through and turn brownish.

NUTRITION: Calories: 255 Cal Fat: 7 g Protein: 15.9 g Carbs: 34. G Fiber: 2.6 g

61. Parsley 'n Lemon Kidney Beans

Preparation Time: 10 Minutes

Cooking Time: 0 Minute

Servings: 6

INGREDIENTS:

- ¼ cup lemon juice (about 1 ½ lemons)
- ¼ cup olive oil
- ¾ cup chopped fresh parsley
- ¾ teaspoon salt

- 1 can (15 ounces) chickpeas, rinsed and drained
- 1 medium cucumber, peeled, seeded and diced
- 1 small red onion, diced
- 2 cans (15 ounces each) red kidney beans, rinsed and drained
- 2 stalks celery, sliced in half or thirds lengthwise and chopped
- 2 tablespoons chopped fresh dill or mint
- 3 cloves garlic, pressed or minced
- Small pinch red pepper flakes

DIRECTIONS:

1. Whisk well in a small bowl the pepper flakes, salt, garlic, and lemon juice until emulsified.
2. In a serving bowl, combine the prepared kidney beans, chickpeas, onion, celery, cucumber, parsley and dill (or mint).
3. Drizzle salad with the dressing and toss well to coat.
4. Serve and enjoy.

NUTRITION: Calories 345 Fat: 11g Carbohydrates: 47g Protein: 16g Fiber: 15g

62. Roasted Vegetables with Polenta

Preparation Time: 5 minutes

Cooking Time: 25 minutes

Servings: 6

INGREDIENTS:

- 2 tsp oregano
- 10 ripe olives, chopped
- 6 dry-packed sun-dried tomatoes, soaked in water to rehydrate, drained and chopped
- 2 plum or Roma tomatoes, sliced
- 10-oz frozen spinach, thawed
- ¼ tsp cracked black pepper

- 2 tsp trans-free margarine
- 1 ½ cups coarse polenta
- 6 cups water
- 2 tbsp. + 1 tsp extra virgin olive oil
- 1 sweet red pepper, seeded, cored and cut into chunks
- 6 medium mushrooms, sliced
- 1 small green zucchini, cut into ¼-inch slices
- 1 small yellow zucchini, cut into ¼-inch slices
- 1 small eggplant, peeled and cut into ¼-inch slices

DIRECTIONS:

1. Grease a baking sheet and a 12-inch circle baking dish, position oven rack 4-inches away from heat source and preheat broiler.
2. With 1 tbsp. olive oil, brush red pepper, mushrooms, zucchini and eggplant. Place in prepared baking sheet in a single layer. Pop in the broiler and broil under low setting.
3. Turn and brush again with oil the veggies after 5 minutes. Continue broiling until veggies are slightly browned and tender.
4. Wash and drain spinach. Set aside.
5. Preheat oven to 350oF.
6. Bring water to a boil in a medium saucepan.
7. Whisk in polenta and lower fire to a simmer. For 5 minutes, cook and stir.
8. Once polenta no longer sticks to pan, add 1/8 tsp pepper and margarine. Mix well and turn off fire.
9. Evenly spread polenta on base of prepped baking dish. Brush tops with olive oil and for ten minutes bake in the oven.
10. When done, remove polenta from oven and keep warm.
11. With paper towels remove excess water from spinach. Layer spinach on top of polenta followed by sliced tomatoes, olives, sun-dried tomatoes, and roasted veggies. Season with remaining pepper and bake for another 10 minutes.
12. Remove from oven, cut into equal servings and enjoy.

NUTRITION: Calories 135 Fat 2g Carbohydrates: 27g Protein 5g Fiber: 6g

63. **Broccoli-Sesame Stir-Fry**

Preparation Time: 10 Minutes

Cooking Time: 8 Minutes

Servings: 4

INGREDIENTS:

- 2 tablespoons extra-virgin olive oil
- 1 teaspoon sesame oil
- 4 cups broccoli florets
- 1 tablespoon grated fresh ginger
- ¼teaspoon sea salt
- 2 garlic cloves, minced
- 2 ablespoons toasted sesame seeds

DIRECTIONS:

1. In a large nonstick skillet over medium-high heat, heat the olive oil and sesame oil until they shimmer.
2. Add the broccoli, ginger, and salt. Cook for 5 to 7 minutes, stirring frequently, until the broccoli begins to brown.
3. Add the garlic. Cook for 30 seconds, stirring constantly.
4. Remove from the heat and stir in the sesame seeds.

NUTRITION: Calories: 134 Fat: 11g Carbohydrates: 9g Sugar: 2g

64. **Creamy Cauliflower Parsnip Mash**

Preparation Time: 4 minutes

Cooking Time: 25 minutes

Servings: 5

INGREDIENTS:

- 1 Medium-Sized Cauliflower
- 2 Parsnips
- 2 Tbsp. Extra Virgin Olive Oil
- 1/2 Tbsp. Salt
- 1/2 Tbsp. Lemon Juice
- 1 Tbsp. Black Pepper
- 5/6 Roasted Garlic Cloves

DIRECTIONS:

1. Cut the vegetables into small pieces.
2. Boil them for 10 to 15 minutes in medium temperature until fork-tender.
3. Drain the water and mash them in a blender.
4. Add the remaining ingredients with the mash and blend until the mixture is smooth as butter.
5. Add water and add salt if needed making sure that the batter isn't too thick or runny and serve.

NUTRITION: Calories: 72 kcal Carbohydrates: 12 g Fat: 0.8 g Protein: 3.7 g

65. Stir-Fried Garlic Chili Beef

Preparation Time: 5 Minutes

Cooking Time: 10 Minutes

Servings: 2

INGREDIENTS:

- 200g Beef Fillet (Sliced)
- 150g Gai Lan (Cut)
- 1 Medium Red Chilli (Seeded, Chopped)
- 1 Tbsp. Sesame Oil
- 4 Large Garlic Cloves (Chopped)
- Soy Sauce
- Toasted Sesame Oil
- Chinese Five-Spice

DIRECTIONS:

1. Season the beef with soy sauce and spices.

2. Stir-fry garlic in sesame oil before adding the beef.
3. Add the gai lan and chili, frying until wilted.
4. Serve with drizzles of light soy sauce, salt, and sesame oil.

NUTRITION: Calories: 192 kcal, Carbohydrates: 2 g, Fat: 8 g Protein: 29 g

66. Pea Stew

Preparation Time: 10 minutes

Cooking time: 25 minutes

Servings: 4

INGREDIENTS:

- 1 carrot, cubed
- 1 yellow onion, chopped
- 1 and ½ tablespoons essential extra virgin olive oil
- 1 celery stick, chopped
- 5 garlic cloves, minced
- 2 cups yellow peas
- 1 and ½ teaspoons cumin, ground
- 1 teaspoon sweet paprika
- ¼ teaspoon chili powder
- A pinch of black pepper
- ¼ teaspoon cinnamon powder
- ½ cup tomatoes, chopped
- Juice of ½ lemon
- 1-quart low-sodium veggie stock
- 1 tablespoon chives, chopped

DIRECTIONS:

1. Heat up a pot using the oil over medium heat, add carrots, onion and celery, stir and cook for 5-6 minutes.
2. Add garlic, peas, cumin, paprika, chili powder, pepper, cinnamon, and tomatoes, fresh lemon juice, peas and stock, stir, bring to many simmers, cook over medium heat for twenty or so minutes, add chives, toss, divide into bowls and serve.

3. Enjoy!

NUTRITION: Calories: 272 Cal Fat: 6 g Fiber: 7 g Carbs: 14 g Protein: 9 g

67. Feta Frittata & Spinach

Preparation Time: 15 minutes

Cooking Time: 10 minutes

Servings: 4

INGREDIENTS:

- ½ small brown onion
- 250g baby spinach
- ½ cup fcta cheese
- 1 tbsp garlic paste
- 4 beaten eggs

Seasoning Mix

- Salt & Pepper according to taste
- 1 tbsp olive oil

DIRECTIONS:

1. Add finely chop an onion in oil and cook it on medium flame.
2. Add spinach in light brown onions and toss it for 2 min.
3. In eggs, add the mixture of cold spinach and onions.
4. Now add garlic paste, salt, and pepper and mix the mixture.
5. Cook this mixture on low flame and stir eggs gently.
6. Add feta cheese on the eggs and place the pan under the already preheat grill.
7. Cook it almost for 2 to 3 minutes until the frittata is brown.
8. Serve this feta frittata hot or cold.

NUTRITION: Calories: 210 Carbs: 5g Fat: 14g Protein: 21g

68. Coconut Green Curry with Boil Rice

Preparation Time: 15 minutes

Cooking Time: 20 minutes

Servings: 8

INGREDIENTS:

- 2tbsp Olive oil
- 12ounces of Tofu
- 2 medium sweet potatoes (cut into cubes)
- Salt-to-taste
- 314ounces Coconut milk
- 4tbsp Green curry paste
- 3 Cups of Broccoli Florets

DIRECTIONS:

1. Remove excess water from tofu and fry it on medium flame. Add salt in it and fry it for 12 minutes.
2. Cook coconut milk, green curry paste, and sweet potato on medium heat and simmer it for 5 mins.
3. Now add broccoli and tofu in it and cook it almost 5 minutes until the broccoli color changes.
4. Serve this coconut and green curry with a handful of boil rice and many raisins on top of it.

NUTRITION: Calories: 170 Carbs: 34g Fat: 2g Protein: 3g

69. Chicken Salad with Chinese Touch

Preparation Time: 15 minutes

Cooking Time: 25 minutes

Servings: 3

INGREDIENTS:

- 1 Medium green onion (thinly sliced)
- 2 Boneless chicken breasts
- 2tbsp Soya sauce

- ¼ Teaspoon white pepper
- 1tbsp sesame oil
- 4 cups romaine lettuce (chopped)
- 1 cup cabbage (shredded)
- ¼ Cup small cubes carrots
- ¼ Cup thin sliced almonds
- ¼ Cup noodles (only for serving)

For Preparing Chinese Dressing:

- 1 Minced garlic clove
- 1 Teaspoon soy sauce
- 1tbsp sesame oil
- 2tbsp Rice vinegar
- 1tbsp Sugar

DIRECTIONS:

1. Prepare Chinese dressing by whisking all ingredients in a bowl.
2. In a bowl, marinate chicken breasts with garlic, olive oil, soy sauce, and white pepper for 20 minutes.
3. Place baking dish in the preheated oven (at 225C).
4. Place chicken breasts in the baking dish and bake it almost for 20 minutes.
5. For assembling the salad, combine romaine lettuce, cabbage, carrots, and green onion.
6. For serving, place a chicken piece in a plate and salad on top of it. Pour some dressing over it alongside noodles.

NUTRITION: Calories: 130 Carbs: 10g Fat: 6g Protein: 10g

70. <u>Lentil Soup with Spices</u>

Preparation Time: 15 minutes

Cooking Time: 25 minutes

Servings: 5

INGREDIENTS:

- 1 Cup of yellow onion (cut into cubes)
- 1 Cup of carrot (cut into cubes)
- 1 Cup of turnip
- 2tbsp extra-virgin olive oil
- 2tbsp balsamic vinegar
- 4 cups of baby spinach
- 2 cups brown lentils
- ¼ Cup of fresh parsley

DIRECTIONS:

1. Preheat the pressure cooker on medium flame and add olive oil and vegetables in it.
2. After 5 minutes, add broth, lentils, and salt in the pot and simmer for 15 minutes.
3. Remove the lid and add spinach and vinegar in it.
4. Stir the soup for 5 minutes and turn off the flame.
5. Garnish it with fresh parsley.

NUTRITION: Calories: 96 Carbs: 16g Fat: 1g Protein: 4g

71. <u>Baked Sweet Potato with Red Tahini Sauce</u>

Preparation Time: 15 minutes

Cooking Time: 30 minutes

Servings: 4

INGREDIENTS:

- 15-ounces Canned Chickpeas
- 4 Medium-sized sweet potatoes
- ½ tbsp Olive oil
- 1 Pinch salt
- 1tbsp Lime juice
- 1/2 tbsp of cumin, coriander, and paprika powder

For Garlic Herb Sauce

- ¼ Cup tahini sauce
- ½ tbsp Lime Juice
- 3 cloves garlic
- Salt to taste

DIRECTIONS:

1. Preheat the oven at 204°C. Toss chickpeas in salt, spices & olive oil. Spread them on the foil sheet.
2. Brush sweet potato thin wedges with oil and place them on marinated beans and bake.
3. For the sauce, mix all fixings in a bowl. Add some water in it, but keep it thick.
4. Remove sweet potatoes from the oven after 25 minutes.
5. Garnish this baked sweet potato chickpea salad with hot garlic sauce.

NUTRITION: Calories: 90 Carbs: 20g Fat: 0g Protein: 2g

72. **Bake chicken Top-up with Olives, Tomatoes, and Basil**

Preparation Time: 15 minutes

Cooking Time: 45 minutes

Servings: 4

INGREDIENTS:

- 8 Chicken thighs
- Small Italian tomatoes
- 1tbsp Black pepper & salt
- 1tbsp Olive oil
- 15 Basil leaves (large)
- Small black olives
- 1-2 Fresh red chili flakes

Directions:

1. Marinate chicken pieces with all spices & olive oil and leave it for some time.
2. Assemble chicken pieces in a rimmed pan with top-up with tomatoes, basil leaves, olives, and chili flakes.
3. Bake this chicken in an already preheated oven (at 220C) for 40 minutes.
4. Bake until the chicken is tender, tomatoes, basil, and olives are cooked.
5. Garnish it with fresh parsley and lemon zest.

NUTRITION: Calories: 304 Carbs: 18g Fat: 7g Protein: 41g

73. **Sweet Potato & Chicken Soup with Lentil**

Preparation Time: 15 minutes

Cooking Time: 35 minutes

Servings: 6

INGREDIENTS:

- 10 Celery stalks
- 1 Home-cooked or rotisserie chicken
- 2 medium sweet potatoes
- 5-ounces French lentils
- 2tbsp Fresh lime juice
- ½ head bite-size escarole
- 6 thin-sliced garlic cloves
- ½ Cup dill (finely chop)
- 1tbsp Kosher Salt
- 2tbsp Extra virgin oil

Directions:

1. Add salt, chicken carcass, lentil, and sweet potatoes in 8 ounces of water and boil it on high flame.
2. Cook these items almost for 10-12 minutes and skim off all the foam form on it.

3. Cook garlic and celery in oil almost for 10 minutes until it is tender & light brown, then add shredded roast chicken in it.

4. Add this mixture in the escarole soup and continuously stir it for 5 minutes on medium heat.

5. Add lemon juice and stir in dill. Serve season hot soup with salt.

NUTRITION: Calories: 310 Carbs: 45g Fat: 11g Protein: 13g

74. White Bean Chicken with Winter Green Vegetables

Preparation Time: 15 minutes

Cooking Time: 45 minutes

Servings: 8

INGREDIENTS:

- 4 Garlic cloves
- 1tbsp Olive oil
- 3 medium parsnips
- 1kg Small cubes of chicken
- 1 Teaspoon cumin powder
- 2 Leaks & 1 Green part
- 2 Carrots (cut into cubes)
- 1 ¼ White kidney beans (overnight soaked)
- ½ Teaspoon dried oregano
- 2 Teaspoon Kosher salt
- Cilantro leaves
- 1 1/2tbsp Ground ancho chilies

DIRECTIONS:

1. Cook garlic, leeks, chicken, and olive oil in a large pot on a medium flame for 5 minutes.

2. Now add carrots and parsnips, and after stirring for 2 minutes, add all seasoning ingredients.

3. Stir until the fragrant starts coming from it.

4. Now add beans and 5 cups of water in the pot.

5. Bring it to a boil and reduce the flame.

6. Allow it to simmer almost for 30 minutes and garnish with parsley and cilantro leaves.

NUTRITION: Calories: 263 Carbs: 24g Fat: 7g Protein: 26g

75. Garlic Shrimps with Gritted Cauliflower

Preparation Time: 15 minutes

Cooking Time: 15 minutes

Servings: 2

INGREDIENTS:

For Preparing Shrimps

- 1 Pound Shrimps
- 2-3tbsp Cajun seasoning
- Salt
- 1tbsp Butter/Ghee

For Preparing Cauliflower Grits

- 2tbsp Ghee
- 12-Ounces of Cauliflower
- 1 Garlic clove
- Salt-to-taste

DIRECTIONS:

1. Boil cauliflower and garlic in 8ounces of water on medium flame until it's tender.

2. Blend tender cauliflower in the food processor with ghee. Add steaming water gradually for the right consistency.

3. Sprinkle 2tbsp of Cajun seasoning on shrimps and marinate.

4. In a large skillet, take 3tbsp of ghee and cook shrimps on medium flame.

5. Place a large spoon of cauliflower grits in bowl top up with fried shrimps.

NUTRITION: Calories: 107 Carbs: 1g Fat: 3g Protein: 20g

76. Garlic & Squash Noodles

Preparation Time: 15 minutes

Cooking Time: 15 minutes

Servings: 4

INGREDIENTS:

For Preparing Sauce

- ¼ Cup coconut milk
- 6 Large dates
- 2/3g Gritted coconut
- 6 Garlic cloves
- 2tbsp Ginger paste
- 2tbsp Red curry paste

For Preparing Noodles

- 1 Large boil squash noodles
- ½ Julienne cut carrots
- ½ Julienne cut zucchini
- 1 small red bell pepper
- ¼ Cup cashew nuts

DIRECTIONS:

1. For making sauce, blend all the ingredients and make a thick puree.
2. Cut spaghetti squash lengthwise and make noodles.
3. Lightly brush the baking tray with olive oil and bake squash noodles at 40C for 5-6 minutes.
4. For serving, incorporate noodles and puree in a bowl. Or serve puree alongside the noodles.

NUTRITION: Calories: 405 Carbs: 107g Fat: 28g Protein: 7g

77. Garlic Chicken Bake with Basil &Tomatoes

Preparation Time: 15 minutes

Cooking Time: 30 minutes

Servings: 4

INGREDIENTS:

- ½ medium yellow onion
- 2tbsp Olive oil
- 3 Minced Garlic Cloves
- 1 Cup Basil (loosely cut)
- 1.lb Boneless chicken breast
- 14.5-ounces Italian chop tomatoes
- Salt & pepper
- 4 Medium zucchinis (spiralized into noodles)
- 1tbsp crushed red pepper
- 2tbsp Olive oil

DIRECTIONS:

1. Pound the chicken pieces with a pan for fast cooking. Sprinkle salt, pepper, and oil on chicken pieces and marinate both sides of chicken equally.
2. Fry chicken pieces on a large hot skillet for 2-3 minutes on each side.
3. Sautee onion in the same skillet pan until it's brown. Add tomatoes, basil leaves, and garlic in it.
4. Simmer it for 3 minutes and add all spices and chicken in the skillet.
5. Serve it on the plate along with saucy zoodles.

NUTRITION: Calories: 44 Carbs: 7g Fat: 0g Protein: 2g

78. Smoked Trout Wrapped in Lettuce

Preparation Time: 15 minutes

Cooking Time: 45 minutes

Servings: 4

INGREDIENTS:

- ¼ Cup salt-roasted potatoes
- 1 cup grape tomatoes
- ½ Cup basil leaves
- 16 small & medium size lettuce leaves
- 1/3 cup Asian sweet chili
- 2 Carrots
- 1/3 Cup Shallots (thin sliced)
- ¼ Cup thin slice Jalapenos
- 1tbsp Sugar
- 2-4.5 Ounces skinless smoked trout
- 2tbsp Fresh lime Juice
- 1 Cucumber

DIRECTIONS:

1. Cut carrots and cucumber in slim strip size.
2. Marinate these vegetables for 20 mins with sugar, fish sauce, lime juice, shallots, and jalapeno.
3. Add trout pieces and other herbs in this vegetable mixture and blend.
4. Strain water from vegetable and trout mixture and again toss it to blend.
5. Place lettuce leaves on a plate and transfer trout salad on them.
6. Garnish this salad with peanuts and chili sauce.

NUTRITION: Calories: 180 Carbs: 0g Fat: 12g Protein: 18g

79. <u>Crusted Salmon with Walnuts & Rosemary</u>

Preparation Time: 15 minutes

Cooking Time: 20 minutes

Servings: 6

INGREDIENTS:

- 1 Mince garlic clove

- 1tbsp Dijon mustard
- ¼ tbsp Lemon zest
- 1tbsp Lemon juice
- 1tbsp fresh rosemary
- 1/2 tbsp Honey
- Olive oil
- Fresh parsley
- 3tbsp Chopped walnuts
- 1 Pound skinless salmon
- 1tbsp Fresh crushed red pepper
- Salt & pepper
- Lemon wedges for garnish
- 3tbsp Panko breadcrumbs
- 1tbsp extra-virgin olive oil

DIRECTIONS:

1. Spread the baking sheet in the oven and preheat it at 240C.
2. In a bowl, mix mustard paste, garlic, salt, olive oil, honey, lemon juice, crushed red pepper, rosemary, pus honey.
3. Combine panko, walnuts, and oil and spread thin fish slice on the baking sheet. Spray olive oil equally on both sides of the fish.
4. Place walnut mixture on the salmon with the mustard mixture on top it.
5. Bake the salmon almost for 12 minutes. Garnish it with fresh parsley and lemon wedges and serve it hot.

NUTRITION: Calories: 227 Carbs: 0g Fat: 12g Protein: 29g

80. <u>Roasted Vegetables with Sweet Potatoes and White Beans</u>

Preparation Time: 15 minutes

Cooking Time: 25 minutes

Servings: 4

INGREDIENTS:

- 2 small sweet potatoes, dice
- ½ red onion, cut into ¼-inch dice
- 1 medium carrot, peeled and thinly sliced
- 4 ounces green beans, trimmed
- ¼ cup extra-virgin olive oil
- 1 teaspoon salt
- ¼ teaspoon freshly ground black pepper
- 1 (15½-ounce) can white beans, drained and rinsed
- 1 tablespoon minced or grated lemon zest
- 1 tablespoon chopped fresh dill

DIRECTIONS:

1. Preheat the oven to 400°F.
2. Combine the sweet potatoes, onion, carrot, green beans, oil, salt, and pepper on a large rimmed baking sheet and mix to combine well. Arrange in a single layer.
3. Roast until the vegetables are tender, 20 to 25 minutes.
4. Add the white beans, lemon zest, and dill, mix well and serve.

NUTRITION: Calories: 315 Total Fat: 13g Total Carbohydrates: 42g Sugar: 5g Fiber: 13g Protein: 10g Sodium: 632mg

81. Roasted Tofu And Greens

Preparation Time: 10 minutes

Cooking Time: 20 minutes

Servings: 4

INGREDIENTS:

- 3 cups baby spinach or kale
- 1 tablespoon sesame oil
- 1 tablespoon ginger, minced

- 1 garlic clove, minced
- 1-pound firm tofu, cut into 1-inch dice
- 1 tablespoon gluten-free tamari or soy sauce
- ¼ teaspoon red pepper flakes (optional)
- 1 teaspoon rice vinegar
- 2 scallions, thinly sliced

DIRECTIONS:

1. Preheat the oven to 400°F.
2. Combine the spinach, oil, ginger, and garlic on a large rimmed baking sheet.
3. Bake until the spinach has wilted, 3 to 5 minutes.
4. Add the tofu, tamari, and red pepper flakes (if using) and toss to combine well.
5. Bake until the tofu is beginning to brown, 10 to 15 minutes.
6. Top with the vinegar and scallions and serve.

NUTRITION: Calories: 121 Total Fat: 8g Total Carbohydrates: 4g Sugar: 1g Fiber: 2g Protein: 10g Sodium: 258mg

82. Tofu and Italian-Seasoned Summer Vegetables

Preparation Time: 10 minutes

Cooking Time: 20 minutes

Servings: 4

INGREDIENTS:

- 2 large zucchinis, cut into ¼-inch slices
- 2 large summer squash, cut into ¼-inch-thick slices
- 1-pound firm tofu, cut into 1-inch dice
- 1 cup vegetable broth or water
- 3 tablespoons extra-virgin olive oil
- 2 garlic cloves, sliced

- 1 teaspoon salt
- 1 teaspoon Italian herb seasoning blend
- ¼ teaspoon freshly ground black pepper
- 1 tablespoon thinly sliced fresh basil

DIRECTIONS:

1. Preheat the oven to 400°F.
2. Combine the zucchini, squash, tofu, broth, oil, garlic, salt, Italian herb seasoning blend, and pepper on a large rimmed baking sheet, and mix well.
3. Roast within 20 minutes.
4. Sprinkle with the basil and serve.

NUTRITION: Calories: 213 Total Fat: 16g Total Carbohydrates: 9g Sugar: 4g Fiber: 3g Protein: 13g Sodium: 806mg

83. **Spiced Broccoli, Cauliflower, And Tofu With Red Onion**

Preparation Time: 10 minutes

Cooking Time: 25 minutes

Servings: 2

INGREDIENTS:

- 2 cups broccoli florets
- 2 cups cauliflower florets
- 1 medium red onion, diced
- 3 tablespoons extra-virgin olive oil
- 1 teaspoon salt
- ¼ teaspoon freshly ground black pepper
- 1-pound firm tofu, cut into 1-inch dice
- 1 garlic clove, minced
- 1 (¼-inch) piece fresh ginger, minced

DIRECTIONS:

1. Preheat the oven to 400°F.

2. Combine the broccoli, cauliflower, onion, oil, salt, and pepper on a large rimmed baking sheet, and mix well.
3. Roast until the vegetables have softened, 10 to 15 minutes.
4. Add the tofu, garlic, and ginger. Roast within 10 minutes.
5. Gently mix the ingredients on the baking sheet to combine the tofu with the vegetables and serve.

NUTRITION: Calories: 210 Total Fat: 15g Total Carbohydrates: 11g Sugar: 4g Fiber: 4g Protein: 12g Sodium: 626mg

84. **Tempeh And Root Vegetable Bake**

Preparation Time: 10 minutes

Cooking Time: 30 minutes

Servings: 4

INGREDIENTS:

- 1 tablespoon extra-virgin olive oil
- 1 large sweet potato, dice
- 2 carrots, thinly sliced
- 1 fennel bulb, trimmed and cut into ¼-inch dice
- 2 teaspoons minced fresh ginger
- 1 garlic clove, minced
- 12 ounces tempeh, cut into ½-inch dice
- ½ cup vegetable broth
- 1 tablespoon gluten-free tamari or soy sauce
- 2 scallions, thinly sliced

DIRECTIONS:

1. Preheat the oven to 400°F. Grease a baking sheet with the oil.

2. Arrange the sweet potato, carrots, fennel, ginger, and garlic in a single layer on the baking sheet.

3. Bake until the vegetables have softened, about 15 minutes.

4. Add the tempeh, broth, and tamari.

5. Bake again until the tempeh is heated through and lightly browned 10 to 15 minutes.

6. Add the scallions, mix well, and serve.

NUTRITION: Calories: 276 Total Fat: 13g Total Carbohydrates: 26g Sugar: 5g Fiber: 4g Protein: 19g Sodium: 397mg

SMOOTHIE AND DRINKS

85. Mango and Cherries Smoothie

Preparation time: 5 minutes

Cooking time: 0 minutes

Servings: 4

INGREDIENTS:

- 1 cup cherries, pitted
- 1 mango, peeled, chopped
- 1 cup of water
- 1 teaspoon dried mint
- 1 orange, peeled, chopped

DIRECTIONS:

1. Put all ingredients in the blender.
2. Blend the smoothie until it is smooth and pour in the glasses.

NUTRITION: 87 calories,1.4g protein, 21.5g carbohydrates, 0.4g fat, 3g fiber, 0mg cholesterol, 5mg sodium, 227mg potassium.

86. Cayenne Pepper Smoothie

Preparation time: 5 minutes

Cooking time: 0 minutes

Servings: 4

INGREDIENTS:

- 1 teaspoon cayenne pepper
- 1 avocado, chopped
- ½ cup fresh spinach, chopped
- 1 cup of water
- 2 tablespoons coconut shred
- 1 cup of coconut milk

DIRECTIONS:

1. Blend cayenne pepper, avocado, spinach, water, coconut shred, and coconut milk until smooth.

NUTRITION: 268 calories,2.5g protein, 9g carbohydrates, 26.7g fat, 5.4g fiber, 0mg cholesterol, 18mg sodium, 432mg potassium.

87. Turmeric Smoothie

Preparation time: 5 minutes

Cooking time: 0 minutes

Servings: 2

INGREDIENTS:

- 1 tablespoon ground turmeric
- 1 cup of coconut milk
- 2 bananas, chopped
- 1 tablespoon fresh lemon juice

DIRECTIONS:

1. Put all ingredients in the blender.
2. Blend the smoothie well.

NUTRITION: 395 calories,4.4g protein, 36g carbohydrates, 29.4g fat, 6.5g fiber, 0mg cholesterol, 22mg sodium, 833mg potassium.

88. Tahini Smoothie

Preparation time: 5 minutes

Cooking time: 0 minutes

Servings: 4

INGREDIENTS:

- 2 tablespoons tahini paste
- 4 bananas, chopped
- 2 oranges, chopped
- ½ cup of water

DIRECTIONS:

1. Blend the ingredients in the blender.
2. When the mixture is smooth, pour it in the glasses.

NUTRITION: 193 calories,3.4g protein, 39.4g carbohydrates, 4.5g fat, 6g fiber, 0mg cholesterol, 11mg sodium, 620mg potassium.

89. Herbal Tea

Preparation time: 15 minutes

Cooking time: 10 minutes

Servings: 4

INGREDIENTS:

- 2 tablespoons herbal tea
- 1 orange, sliced
- 4 cups of water

DIRECTIONS:

1. Bring the water to boil.
2. Then remove it from the oven and add herbal tea and oranges.
3. Leave the tea for 15 minutes.

NUTRITION: 22 calories, 0.4g protein, 5.4g carbohydrates, 0.1g fat, 1.1g fiber, 0mg cholesterol, 7mg sodium, 86mg potassium.

90. Water with Herbs

Preparation time: 25 minutes

Cooking time: 0 minutes

Servings: 4

INGREDIENTS:

- 1 teaspoon rosemary
- 1 teaspoon mint
- 1 teaspoon chamomile
- 4 cups of water
- ½ lime

DIRECTIONS:

1. Pour water in the bottle.
2. Add all remaining ingredients and leave the drink for 15-20 minutes.

NUTRITION: 4 calories, 0.1g protein, 1.1g carbohydrates, 0.1g fat, 0.4g fiber, 0mg cholesterol, 8mg sodium, 16mg potassium.

91. Green Tea

Preparation time: 15 minutes

Cooking time: 10 minutes

Servings: 4

INGREDIENTS:

- 4 teaspoons green tea
- 1 tablespoon fresh mint
- 1 tablespoon lemon juice
- 4 cups of water

DIRECTIONS:

1. Bring the water to boil and add green tea.
2. Leave the tea for 10 minutes.
3. Then add mint and lemon juice.

NUTRITION: 2 calories, 0.1g protein, 0.2g carbohydrates, 0g fat, 0.1g fiber, 0mg cholesterol, 8mg sodium, 14mg potassium.

92. Ginger Tea

Preparation time: 15 minutes

Cooking time: 15 minutes

Servings: 4

INGREDIENTS:

- 2 tablespoons ground ginger
- ½ lemon
- 5 cups of water
- 1 oz cranberries
- 1 tablespoon liquid honey

DIRECTIONS:

1. Bring the water to boil.
2. Add cranberries, ground ginger, and juice from ½ of lemon.
3. Simmer the tea for 5 minutes.
4. Then add honey.

NUTRITION: 31 calories, 0.4g protein, 7.6g carbohydrates, 0.2g fat, 0.8g fiber, 0mg cholesterol, 10mg sodium, 64mg potassium.

93. Cinnamon Tea

Preparation time: 15 minutes

Cooking time: 15 minutes

Servings: 4

INGREDIENTS:

- 2 tablespoons green tea
- 4 cups of water
- 1 teaspoon ground cinnamon

DIRECTIONS:

1. Bring water to boil.
2. Add green tea and stir the drink.
3. Then add ground cinnamon and pour it in the cups.

NUTRITION: 1 calorie, 0g protein, 0.5g carbohydrates, 0g fat, 0.3g fiber, 0mg cholesterol, 7mg sodium, 12mg potassium.

94. Berries Tea

Preparation time: 15 minutes

Cooking time: 15 minutes

Servings: 4

INGREDIENTS:

- 2 tablespoons black tea
- 1 cup blueberries
- 5 cups of water

DIRECTIONS:

1. Bring the water to boil. Add blueberries. Simmer the mixture for 5 minutes.
2. Then blend the mixture, add black tea, and remove the drink from the heat.
3. Pour the drink in the cups.

NUTRITION: 21 calories, 0.3g protein, 5.3g carbohydrates, 0.1g fat, 0.9g fiber, 0mg cholesterol, 9mg sodium, 34mg potassium.

95. Green Tea with Lemon

Preparation time: 5 minutes

Cooking time: 15 minutes

Servings: 4

INGREDIENTS:

- 4 teaspoons green tea
- 4 lemon slices

- 4 cups of water

DIRECTIONS:

1. Bring the water to boil. Add green tea and remove the drink from the heat.
2. Then add lemon slices and pour the drink in the cups.

NUTRITION: 2 calories, 0.1g protein, 0.7g carbohydrates, 0g fat, 0.2g fiber, 0mg cholesterol, 7mg sodium, 27mg potassium.

96. Coconut Late

Preparation time: 5 minutes

Cooking time: 10 minutes

Servings: 4

INGREDIENTS:

- 4 teaspoons ground coffee
- 2 cups of coconut milk
- 1 cup of water
- 1 tablespoon shredded coconut

DIRECTIONS:

1. Bring the water to boil.
2. Add ground coffee and mix well.
3. Then pour the liquid in the glasses.
4. Add coconut milk and shredded coconut.

NUTRITION: 280 calories, 2.8g protein, 6.8g carbohydrates, 29g fat, 2.8g fiber, 0mg cholesterol, 20mg sodium, 323mg potassium.

97. Apple Tea

Preparation time: 10 minutes

Cooking time: 10 minutes

Servings: 4

INGREDIENTS:

- 4 lime slices
- 4 cups of water
- 1 cup apple, chopped

DIRECTIONS:

1. Pour water in the pan. Add lime and apple.

2. Simmer the apple tea for 10 minutes.

NUTRITION: 30 calories, 0.2g protein, 8.1g carbohydrates, 0.1g fat, 1.4g fiber, 0mg cholesterol, 8mg sodium, 65mg potassium.

98. Pears Chai

Preparation time: 5 minutes

Cooking time: 10 minutes

Servings: 4

INGREDIENTS:

- 1 tablespoon chai
- 4 pears, chopped
- 5 cups of water

DIRECTIONS:

1. Mix water with chai and pears.
2. Bring the liquid to boil and simmer for 5-9 minutes.

NUTRITION: 121 calories, 0.8g protein, 31.8g carbohydrates, 0.3g fat, 6.5g fiber, 0mg cholesterol, 11mg sodium, 245mg potassium.

99. Cherry Drink

Preparation time: 5 minutes

Cooking time: 0 minutes

Servings: 4

INGREDIENTS:

- 5 cups of water
- 2 cups cherries
- 1 tablespoon liquid honey

DIRECTIONS:

1. Mix cherries with water and bring to boil.
2. Pour the drink in the glasses and add liquid honey.

NUTRITION: 54 calories, 0.8g protein, 13.8g carbohydrates, 0.3g fat, 1.3g fiber, 0mg cholesterol, 9mg sodium, 140mg potassium.

100. Mint Tea

Preparation time: 10 minutes

Cooking time: 10 minutes

Servings: 4

INGREDIENTS:

- 4 teaspoons black tea
- 4 teaspoons fresh mint
- 4 cups of water

DIRECTIONS:

1. Bring water to boil, add fresh mint.
2. Then remove the liquid from the heat, add black tea and stir well.
3. Pour the tea in the glasses.

NUTRITION: 1 calorie, 0.1g protein, 0g carbohydrates, 0g fat, 0.1g fiber, 0mg cholesterol, 8mg sodium, 13mg potassium.

101. Basil Tea

Preparation time: 10 minutes

Cooking time: 10 minutes

Servings: 4

INGREDIENTS:

- 4 lemon slices
- 1 cup fresh basil
- 4 cups of water

DIRECTIONS:

1. Bring water to boil.
2. Add basil and lemon slices.
3. Leave the tea for 10 minutes to rest.

NUTRITION: 3 calories, 0.3g protein, 0.8g carbohydrates, 0.1g fat, 0.3g fiber, 0mg cholesterol, 7mg sodium, 30mg potassium.

102. Berry Milkshake

Preparation time: 5 minutes

Cooking time: 0 minutes

Servings: 2

INGREDIENTS:

- 1 cup strawberries
- 1 cup blueberries

- 1 cup of coconut milk

DIRECTIONS:

1. Put all ingredients in the blender.
2. Blend the mixture until smooth.
3. Pour the cooked milkshake in the glasses.

NUTRITION: 341 calories,3.8g protein, 22.7g carbohydrates, 29.1g fat, 5.8g fiber, 0mg cholesterol, 19mg sodium, 482mg potassium.

103. Banana Smoothie

Preparation time: 5 minutes

Cooking time: 0 minutes

Servings: 4

INGREDIENTS:

- 1 avocado, chopped
- 4 bananas, chopped
- 1 cup of coconut milk

DIRECTIONS:

1. Put all ingredients in the blender and blend until smooth.
2. Pour the smoothie in the glasses.

NUTRITION: 346 calories,3.6g protein, 34.6g carbohydrates, 24.5g fat, 7.8g fiber, 0mg cholesterol, 13mg sodium, 824mg potassium.

SNACKS

104. Shrimp Bowls

Preparation time: 10 minutes

Cooking time: 0 minutes

Servings: 4

INGREDIENTS:

- 1 pound shrimp, peeled, deveined, and cooked
- 1 cup kalamata olives, pitted and sliced
- 1 cup cherry tomatoes, cubed
- ½ cup basil, chopped
- A pinch of salt and black pepper
- 2 tablespoons lime juice
- 2 teaspoons chili powder

DIRECTIONS:

1. In a bowl, combine the shrimp with the kalamata, tomatoes and the other ingredients, toss well, divide into smaller bowls and serve.

NUTRITION: calories 186, fat 5.8, fiber 2.1, carbs 6.4, protein 26.8

105. Italian Salmon Bowls

Preparation time: 10 minutes

Cooking time: 14 minutes

Servings: 4

INGREDIENTS:

- 1 pound salmon fillets, boneless and cubed
- 2 tablespoons olive oil
- 1 teaspoon Italian seasoning
- 1 teaspoon garlic, minced
- ½ cup kalamata olives, pitted and chopped
- ¼ cup basil, chopped
- Salt and black pepper to the taste

DIRECTIONS:

1. In a bowl, combine the salmon with the oil, the Italian seasoning and the other ingredients, toss, arrange on a baking sheet lined with parchment paper and cook at 400 degrees F for 14 minutes.
2. Divide the salmon into bowls and serve.

NUTRITION: calories 270, fat 7.5, fiber 2, carbs 7, protein 7

106. Avocado and Olives Salsa

Preparation time: 10 minutes

Cooking time: 0 minutes

Servings: 4

INGREDIENTS:

- 2 avocados, peeled, pitted and roughly cubed
- 2 tablespoons olive oil
- 1 cup kalamata olives, pitted and halved
- ½ cup cherry tomatoes, cubed
- Juice of 1 lime
- Salt and black pepper to the taste
- 1 tablespoon basil, chopped

DIRECTIONS:

1. In a bowl, combine the avocados with the lime juice and the other ingredients, toss, divide into small bowls and serve as a snack.

NUTRITION: calories 180, fat 3, fiber 5, carbs 8, protein 6

107. Seafood Bowls

Preparation time: 5 minutes

Cooking time: 10 minutes

Servings: 4

INGREDIENTS:

- 1 pound mussels, debearded and scrubbed
- ½ pound shrimp, peeled and deveined
- 4 scallions, chopped
- 2 garlic cloves, minced
- 1 tablespoon olive oil
- 1 tablespoon lemon juice

DIRECTIONS:

1. Heat up a pan with the oil over medium heat, add the scallions and the garlic and sauté for 2 minutes.
2. Add the rest of the ingredients, toss, cook over medium heat for 8 minutes more, divide into bowls and serve.

NUTRITION: calories 90, fat 4, fiber 5, carbs 5, protein 2

108. <u>Lemon Calamari Mix</u>

Preparation time: 10 minutes

Cooking time: 20 minutes

Servings: 4

INGREDIENTS:

- 1 pound calamari rings
- 2 tablespoons olive oil
- ½ cup chicken stock
- A pinch of cayenne pepper
- A pinch of salt and black pepper
- 1 tablespoons lemon juice
- 1 teaspoon chili powder
- 1 teaspoon cumin, ground
- 1 tablespoon chives, chopped

DIRECTIONS:

1. Heat up a pan with the oil over medium heat, add the calamari, the stock and the

other ingredients, toss, cook for 20 minutes, divide into small bowls and serve.

NUTRITION: calories 155, fat 8, fiber 3, carbs 3, protein 7

109. <u>Lemon Seafood Mix</u>

Preparation time: 10 minutes

Cooking time: 12 minutes

Servings: 4

INGREDIENTS:

- 1 cup calamari rings
- 1 cup clams, scrubbed
- 1 pound shrimp, peeled and deveined
- 1 tablespoon avocado oil
- 1 teaspoon lemon juice
- ½ teaspoon rosemary, dried
- 1 teaspoon chili powder
- ½ cup chicken stock
- Salt and black pepper to the taste
- ½ teaspoon turmeric powder

DIRECTIONS:

1. Heat up a pan with the oil over medium heat, add the shrimp, the calamari rings, the clams and the other ingredients, toss, cook for 12 minutes, arrange on a platter and serve.

NUTRITION: calories 238, fat 8, fiber 3, carbs 10, protein 8

110. <u>Coconut Celery Spread</u>

Preparation time: 10 minutes

Cooking time: 15 minutes

Servings: 4

INGREDIENTS:

- 4 celery stalks
- 3 scallions, chopped

- 1 tablespoon olive oil
- 1 tablespoon lime juice
- ½ teaspoon chili powder
- 1 cup coconut cream
- Salt and black pepper to the taste
- 2 tablespoons parsley, chopped

DIRECTIONS:

1. Heat up a pan with the oil over medium heat, add the scallions and sauté for 2 minutes.
2. Add the celery and the other ingredients, toss, cook over medium heat for 13 minutes more, blend using an immersion blender, divide into bowls and serve s a snack.

NUTRITION: calories 140, fat 10, fiber 3, carbs 6, protein 13

111. **Shrimp Salad**

Preparation time: 5 minutes

Cooking time: 10 minutes

Servings: 4

INGREDIENTS:

- 1-pound shrimp, peeled and deveined
- 2 shallots, chopped
- 1 tablespoon olive oil
- Salt and black pepper to the taste
- 1 teaspoon rosemary, dried
- 2 cups coconut cream
- 1 cup cilantro, chopped

DIRECTIONS:

1. Heat up a pan with the oil over medium heat, add the shallots and sauté for 2 minutes.

2. Add the shrimp and the other ingredients, toss, cook over medium heat for 8 minutes, divide into bowls and serve.

NUTRITION: calories 220, fat 8, fiber 0, carbs 5, protein 12

112. **Fennel Salad**

Preparation time: 10 minutes

Cooking time: 0 minutes

Servings: 4

INGREDIENTS:

- 2 tablespoons olive oil
- 2 fennel bulbs, shredded
- 1 cup kalamata olives, pitted and halved
- 1 tablespoon balsamic vinegar
- A pinch of salt and black pepper
- 2 tablespoons lime juice
- 2 tablespoons parsley, chopped
- 2 tablespoons mint, chopped

DIRECTIONS:

1. In a bowl, mix the fennel with the oil and the other ingredients, toss well, keep in the fridge for 10 minutes, divide into bowls and serve.

NUTRITION: calories 160, fat 7, fiber 2, carbs 7, protein 8

113. **Olives and Mango Salsa**

Preparation time: 10 minutes

Cooking time: 0 minutes

Servings: 4

INGREDIENTS:

- 2 mangoes, peeled and cubed
- 2 oranges, peeled and cut into segments
- ½ cup kalamata olives, pitted and halved
- Juice of 1 orange

- Zest of 1 orange, grated
- Juice of 1 lime
- 2 red chili peppers, chopped
- ½ teaspoon ginger, grated
- A pinch of salt and black pepper
- 1 tablespoon avocado oil
- ¼ cup cilantro, chopped

DIRECTIONS:

1. In a bowl, mix the mangoes with the oranges and the other ingredients, toss, divide into smaller bowls and serve.

NUTRITION: calories 170, fat 3, fiber 5.7, carbs 37.6, protein 2.5

114. Stuffed Salmon Wraps

Preparation time: 10 minutes

Cooking time: 0 minutes

Servings: 4

INGREDIENTS:

- 6 ounces smoked salmon, skinless and thinly sliced
- 1 red bell pepper, cut into strips
- 1 cucumber, cut into strips
- 2 tablespoons coconut cream

DIRECTIONS:

1. Place the smoked salmon slices on a working surface, spread the coconut cream on each, divide the cucumber and the bell pepper strips on each slide, roll and serve as a snack.

NUTRITION: calories 120, fat 6, fiber 6, carbs 12, protein 6

115. Mussels and Quinoa Bowls

Preparation time: 10 minutes

Cooking time: 12 minutes

Servings: 4

INGREDIENTS:

- 1 pound mussels, scrubbed
- 2 cups quinoa, cooked
- ½ cup chicken soup
- 1 teaspoon red pepper flakes, crushed
- 1 teaspoon hot paprika
- 2 garlic cloves, minced
- 2 tablespoons parsley, chopped
- 2 tablespoons avocado oil
- 1 yellow onion, chopped
- A pinch of salt and black pepper

DIRECTIONS:

1. Heat up a pan with the oil over medium heat, add the onion and the garlic and sauté for 2 minutes.
2. Add the mussels, quinoa and the other ingredients, toss, cook over medium heat for 10 minutes more, divide into small bowls and serve.

NUTRITION: calories 150, fat 3, fiber 3, carbs 6, protein 8

116. Tuna Bites

Preparation time: 10 minutes

Cooking time: 10 minutes

Servings: 4

INGREDIENTS:

- 1 pound tuna fillets, boneless, skinless and cubed
- 1 pound shrimp, peeled and deveined
- 2 tablespoons olive oil
- 4 scallions, chopped
- Juice of 1 lime

- 1 teaspoon sweet paprika
- 1 teaspoon turmeric powder
- 2 tablespoons coconut aminos
- A pinch of salt and black pepper

DIRECTIONS:

1. Heat up a pan with the oil over medium heat, add the scallions and sauté for 2 minutes.
2. Add the tuna bites and cook them for 2 minutes on each side.
3. Add the shrimp and the remaining ingredients, toss gently, cook everything for 4 minutes more, arrange everything on a platter and serve.

NUTRITION: calories 210, fat 7, fiber 6, carbs 6, protein 7

117. Berries Salsa

Preparation time: 10 minutes

Cooking time: 0 minutes

Servings: 4

INGREDIENTS:

- 1 pound cherry tomatoes, cubed
- 1 cup blackberries
- ½ cup strawberries
- 2 tablespoons avocado oil
- 4 scallions, chopped
- 2 tablespoons garlic powder
- A pinch of salt and black pepper
- ½ tablespoon mint, chopped
- 1 tablespoon chives, chopped

DIRECTIONS:

1. In a bowl, combine the tomatoes with the blackberries, strawberries and the other ingredients, toss, divide into small bowls and serve really cold.

NUTRITION: calories 60, fat 3, fiber 2, carbs 6, protein 7

118. Tomato Dip

Preparation time: 10 minutes

Cooking time: 12 minutes

Servings: 6

INGREDIENTS:

- 1 pound tomatoes, chopped
- 2 carrots, grated
- 4 ounces coconut cream
- A pinch of salt and black pepper
- 1 teaspoon chili powder
- Cooking spray

DIRECTIONS:

1. In a pan, combine the tomatoes with the carrots and the other ingredients, toss and cook over medium heat for 12 minutes.
2. Blend using an immersion blender, divide into small bowls and serve as a party dip.

NUTRITION: calories 150, fat 4, fiber 6, carbs 14, protein 6

119. Cayenne Shrimp Bowls

Preparation time: 10 minutes

Cooking time: 0 minutes

Servings: 2

INGREDIENTS:

- 2 avocados, halved, pitted and cubed
- ½ pound shrimp, cooked, peeled and deveined
- A pinch of salt and black pepper
- 1 tablespoon lemon juice
- 2 tablespoons olive oil
- 1 teaspoon cayenne pepper
- ½ teaspoon rosemary, dried

- ½ teaspoon oregano, dried

- 1 teaspoon sweet paprika

DIRECTIONS:

1. In a bowl, combine the avocados with the shrimp, salt, pepper and the other ingredients, toss, divide into small bowls and serve.

NUTRITION: calories 160, fat 10, fiber 7, carbs 12, protein 7

120. Masala Radish Wedges

Preparation time: 5 minutes

Cooking time: 25 minutes

Servings: 4

INGREDIENTS:

- 1 pound radishes, cut into wedges

- 2 tablespoons olive oil

- ½ teaspoon garam masala

- ½ teaspoon oregano, dried

- ½ teaspoon basil, dried

- Salt and black pepper to the taste

- 1 tablespoon chives, chopped

DIRECTIONS:

1. Spread the radishes on a baking sheet lined with parchment paper, add the oil, garam masala and the other ingredients, toss and bake at 420 degrees F for 25 minutes.

2. Divide the radish bites into bowls and serve as a snack.

NUTRITION: calories 30, fat 1, fiber 2, carbs 7, protein 1

121. Radish Dip

Preparation time: 5 minutes

Cooking time: 0 minutes

Servings: 4

INGREDIENTS:

- 2 avocados, pitted, peeled and chopped

- 1 cup radishes, chopped

- 1 cup coconut cream

- 4 spring onions, chopped

- 1 tablespoon lemon juice

- A pinch of salt and black pepper

- 1 tablespoon avocado oil

DIRECTIONS:

1. In a blender, combine the avocados with the radishes and the other ingredients, pulse well, divide into bowls and serve as a party dip.

NUTRITION: calories 162, fat 8, fiber 4, carbs 6, protein 6

122. Olives Salsa

Preparation time: 10 minutes

Cooking time: 0 minutes

Servings: 6

INGREDIENTS:

- 1 teaspoon cumin seeds

- 1 tablespoon avocado oil

- 2 oranges, peeled and cut into segments

- 1 cup kalamata olives, pitted and halved

- 1 tablespoon oregano, chopped

- 1 tablespoon chives, chopped

- 1 tablespoon balsamic vinegar

- ½ tablespoon ginger, grated

- ½ teaspoon fennel seeds

DIRECTIONS:

1. In a bowl, combine the oranges with the olives, cumin and the other ingredients, toss, keep in the fridge for 10 minutes, divide into small bowls and serve.

NUTRITION: calories 120, fat 1, fiber 3, carbs 5, protein 9

123. Balsamic Radish Salsa

Preparation time: 5 minutes

Cooking time: 0 minutes

Servings: 4

INGREDIENTS:

- 1 tablespoon olive oil
- 2 red bell peppers, cut into thin strips
- 2 green bell peppers, cut into strips
- 1 cup radishes, cubed
- 2 tablespoons balsamic vinegar
- 1 tablespoon ginger, grated
- 1 teaspoon chili powder
- 1 tablespoon lemon juice
- A pinch of salt and black pepper
- 1 tablespoon basil, chopped

DIRECTIONS:

1. In a bowl, combine the bell peppers with the radishes, the oil and the other ingredients, toss, divide into small bowls and serve as a party salsa.

NUTRITION: calories 107, fat 4, fiber 2, carbs 6, protein 6

124. Coconut Beans Dip

Preparation time: 10 minutes

Cooking time: 20 minutes

Servings: 6

INGREDIENTS:

- 2 cups canned red kidney beans, drained
- 2 tablespoons olive oil
- 1 yellow onion, chopped
- ½ cup chicken stock

- ½ cup coconut cream
- ¼ teaspoon oregano, dried
- ¼ teaspoon garlic powder
- ¼ teaspoon onion powder
- Salt and black pepper to the taste
- 1 tablespoon chives, chopped

DIRECTIONS:

1. Heat up a pan with the oil over medium heat, add the onion and sauté for 5 minutes.
2. Add the stock, oregano and the other ingredients except the cream and the chives, stir, and cook over medium heat for 15 minutes more.
3. Add the cream, blend the mix using an immersion blender, divide into bowls and serve with the chives sprinkled on top.

NUTRITION: calories 302, fat 10.2, fiber 10.2, carbs 40.7, protein 14.6

125. Avocado Dip

Preparation time: 10 minutes

Cooking time: 0 minutes

Servings: 4

INGREDIENTS:

- 2 avocados, pitted, peeled and chopped
- 1 cup cherry tomatoes, chopped
- 1 tablespoon lemon juice
- 2 tablespoons coconut oil
- 1 teaspoon chili powder
- ½ cup mint, chopped
- A pinch of salt and black pepper

DIRECTIONS:

1. In a blender, mix the tomatoes with the avocado and the other ingredients, pulse

well, divide into small bowls and serve as a party dip.

NUTRITION: calories 150, fat 7, fiber 6, carbs 8.8, protein 6

126. <u>Balsamic Shrimp Bowls</u>

Preparation time: 10 minutes

Cooking time: 0 minutes

Servings: 4

INGREDIENTS:

- 2 tablespoons avocado oil
- 4 scallions, chopped
- 1-pound shrimp, cooked, deveined and peeled
- 1 cup watermelon, peeled and cubed
- ½ cup strawberries
- 2 tablespoons lemon juice
- A pinch of cayenne pepper
- 1 tablespoon balsamic vinegar

DIRECTIONS:

1. In a bowl, combine the shrimp with the watermelon, scallions and the other ingredients, toss, divide into smaller bowls and serve.

NUTRITION: calories 205, fat 12, fiber 2, carbs 9, protein 8

127. <u>Cayenne Blackberries Dip</u>

Preparation time: 10 minutes

Cooking time: 0 minutes

Servings: 4

INGREDIENTS:

- 1 avocado, pitted, peeled and chopped
- 1 red chili pepper, minced
- 1 cup blackberries
- ½ cup blueberries
- A pinch of cayenne pepper
- 2 tablespoons lemon juice

DIRECTIONS:

1. In a blender, combine the avocado with the berries and the other ingredients, pulse well, divide into small bowls and serve as a party dip.

NUTRITION: calories 120, fat 2, fiber 2, carbs 7, protein 4

128. <u>Cilantro Crackers</u>

Preparation time: 5 minutes

Cooking time: 25 minutes

Servings: 4

INGREDIENTS:

- 1 cup coconut flour
- A pinch of salt and black pepper
- 1 cup cilantro, chopped
- 1 teaspoon lemon zest, grated
- 1 tablespoon lemon juice
- 2 eggs, whisked
- ½ teaspoon baking powder

DIRECTIONS:

1. In a bowl, mix the flour with the eggs and the other ingredients, and stir well.
2. Spread the mix on a baking sheet lined with parchment paper, cut into triangles and cook at 380 degrees F for 25 minutes.
3. Cool the squares down and serve them as a snack.

NUTRITION: calories 49, fat 2.7, fiber 1.4, carbs 2.8, protein 3.4

DESSERT RECIPES

129. Cherry Jam

Preparation time: 10 minutes

Cooking time: 10 minutes

Servings: 6

INGREDIENTS:

- 3 cups cherries, pitted, chopped
- 2 tablespoons honey

DIRECTIONS:

1. Mix the cherries with honey and sauté the mixture for 10 minutes.
2. Transfer the jam in the glass cans and close the lids.

NUTRITION: 71 calories, 0g protein, 17.8g carbohydrates, 0g fat, 0.5g fiber, 0mg cholesterol, 20mg sodium, 4mg potassium

130. Ginger Mix

Preparation time: 10 minutes

Cooking time: 0 minutes

Servings: 6

INGREDIENTS:

- 3 tablespoons minced ginger
- 1 lemon, minced
- 1 tablespoon liquid honey

DIRECTIONS:

1. Put all ingredients in the can and carefully mix.
2. Close the lid and store the meal in the fridge for up to 7 days.

NUTRITION: 23 calories, 0.4g protein, 5.7g carbohydrates, 0.2g fat, 0.6g fiber, 0mg cholesterol, 1mg sodium, 51mg potassium

131. Mango Sorbet

Preparation time: 40 minutes

Cooking time: 0 minutes

Servings: 4

INGREDIENTS:

- 2 mangoes, peeled and cubed
- ¼ cup of water

DIRECTIONS:

1. Blend the mangoes until smooth and mix with water.
2. Pour the mixture in the plastic vessel and freeze for 40 minutes.
3. Then blend the mixture until smooth and transfer in the serving bowls.

NUTRITION: 101 calories, 1.4g protein, 25.2g carbohydrates, 0.6g fat, 2.7g fiber, 0mg cholesterol, 2mg sodium, 282mg potassium

132. Watermelon Juice

Preparation time: 10 minutes

Cooking time: 15 minutes

Servings: 4

INGREDIENTS:

- 3 cups watermelon
- 1 cup of orange juice

DIRECTIONS:

1. Blend the watermelon until smooth.
2. Then pour the orange juice in the ice mold and freeze until solid.
3. Pour the blended watermelon in the glasses.
4. Add orange juice cubes.

NUTRITION: 62 calories, 1.1g protein, 15g carbohydrates, 0.3g fat, 0.6g fiber, 0mg cholesterol, 2mg sodium, 251mg potassium

133. Orange Ice

Preparation time: 10 minutes

Cooking time: 40 minutes

Servings: 4

INGREDIENTS:

- 4 cups orange juice
- 1 tablespoon liquid honey

DIRECTIONS:

1. Mix orange juice with liquid honey.
2. Then pour the mixture in the ice cube molds and freeze for 40 minutes.
3. Put the orange cubes in the food processor and blend until smooth.

NUTRITION: 128 calories, 1.7g protein, 30.1g carbohydrates, 0.5g fat, 0.5g fiber, 0mg cholesterol, 2mg sodium, 499mg potassium

134. Oatmeal Pudding

Preparation time: 10 minutes

Cooking time: 30 minutes

Servings: 4

INGREDIENTS:

- 2 cups plain yogurt
- 1 cup oatmeal
- 1 teaspoon ground cinnamon
- 2 tablespoons of liquid honey

DIRECTIONS:

1. Mix plain yogurt with oatmeal and ground cinnamon.
2. Leave the mixture for 30 minutes.
3. Then put the pudding in the serving glasses and top with liquid honey.

NUTRITION: 198 calories, 9.7g protein, 31.6g carbohydrates, 2.8g fat, 2.4g fiber, 7mg cholesterol, 87mg sodium, 369mg potassium

135. Peach Pudding

Preparation time: 10 minutes

Cooking time: 10 minutes

Servings: 4

INGREDIENTS:

- 2 cups peaches, pitted, chopped

- 1 cup coconut cream
- 2 tablespoons almond flour
- 1 teaspoon vanilla extract

DIRECTIONS:

1. Bring the coconut cream to boil and add the almond flour.
2. Simmer the liquid for 5 minutes.
3. Then blend the peaches until smooth and add in the coconut cream mixture.
4. Stir well and transfer the pudding in the serving bowls.

NUTRITION: 192 calories, 2.8g protein, 11.2g carbohydrates, 16.2g fat, 2.9g fiber, 0mg cholesterol, 10mg sodium, 302mg potassium

136. Quinoa Pudding

Preparation time: 10 minutes

Cooking time: 10 minutes

Servings: 4

INGREDIENTS:

- 3 cups of coconut milk
- 1 tablespoon almond flour
- 1 cup quinoa
- 2 bananas, chopped
- 1 tablespoon vanilla extract

DIRECTIONS:

1. Mix coconut milk with quinoa and almond flour.
2. Bring the mixture to boil and remove from the heat.
3. Add vanilla extract and bananas.
4. Stir the pudding well.

NUTRITION: 643 calories, 11.1g protein, 51.5g carbohydrates, 46.5g fat, 8.7g fiber, 0mg cholesterol, 31mg sodium, 929mg potassium

137. Chia and Banana Pudding

Preparation time: 10 minutes

Cooking time: 0 minutes

Servings: 3

INGREDIENTS:

- 1 cup coconut cream
- 4 tablespoons chia seeds
- 2 bananas, chopped

DIRECTIONS:

1. Blend the bananas until smooth and mix them with coconut cream and chia seeds.
2. Pour the pudding into the serving bowls.

NUTRITION: 346 calories, 5.8g protein, 30.4g carbohydrates, 25.1g fat, 10.3g fiber, 0mg cholesterol, 16mg sodium, 569mg potassium

138. Strawberry Compote

Preparation time: 10 minutes

Cooking time: 20 minutes

Servings: 6

INGREDIENTS:

- 3 cups strawberries
- 1 cup apricots, chopped
- 2 cups of water

DIRECTIONS:

1. Bring the water to boil and add strawberries.
2. Then add apricots and simmer the meal for 10 minutes.
3. Cool the compote and pour it into glasses.

NUTRITION: 35 calories, 0.8g protein, 8.4g carbohydrates, 0.4g fat, 1.9g fiber, 0mg cholesterol, 3mg sodium, 178mg potassium

139. Blackberry Pudding

Preparation time: 10 minutes

Cooking time: 0 minutes

Servings: 6

INGREDIENTS:

- 3 cups blackberries
- 1 cup coconut cream
- 1 tablespoon chia seeds

DIRECTIONS:

1. Blend the blackberries until smooth and mix them with chia seeds and coconut cream.
2. Pour the pudding in the serving glasses.

NUTRITION: 134 calories, 2.3g protein, 10.1g carbohydrates, 10.6g fat, 5.5g fiber, 0mg cholesterol, 7mg sodium, 231mg potassium

140. Baked Apricot Halves

Preparation time: 10 minutes

Cooking time: 15 minutes

Servings: 4

INGREDIENTS:

- 8 apricots, halved
- 1 teaspoon ground cinnamon
- 1 oz almonds, chopped

DIRECTIONS:

1. Put the apricot halves in the tray in one layer.
2. Top the fruits with ground cinnamon and almonds.
3. Bake the dessert for 15 minutes at 365F.

NUTRITION: 76 calories, 2.4g protein, 9.7g carbohydrates, 4g fat, 2.6g fiber, 0mg cholesterol, 1mg sodium, 236mg potassium

141. Chia Bars

Preparation time: 20 minutes

Cooking time: 0 minutes

Servings: 4

INGREDIENTS:

- 3 oz chia seeds
- 6 dates, chopped
- 3 oz walnuts, chopped
- 1 teaspoon lemon zest, grated
- 1 teaspoon honey

INGREDIENTS:

1. In the mixing bowl, mix chia seeds with dates, walnuts, lemon zest, and honey.
2. Mix the mixture until smooth.
3. Then roll it up in the shape of the square and cut into bars.

NUTRITION: 275 calories, 9g protein, 21.9g carbohydrates, 19.1g fat, 9.8g fiber, 0mg cholesterol, 4mg sodium, 282mg potassium

142. Chocolate Mousse

Preparation time: 10 minutes

Cooking time: 0 minutes

Servings: 4

INGREDIENTS:

- 1 avocado, pitted, peeled, chopped
- 1 tablespoon cocoa powder
- ¼ cup coconut cream

DIRECTIONS:

1. Blend the avocado with cocoa powder.
2. When the mixture is smooth, add coconut cream.
3. Pulse the mousse for 2 minutes more.

NUTRITION: 140 calories, 1.5g protein, 5.9g carbohydrates, 13.6g fat, 4.1g fiber, 0mg cholesterol, 6mg sodium, 317mg potassium

143. Carrot Soufflé

Preparation time: 10 minutes

Cooking time: 25 minutes

Servings: 4

INGREDIENTS:

- 2 cups carrot, grated
- 4 eggs, beaten
- ½ cup coconut cream
- 1 tablespoon liquid honey

DIRECTIONS:

1. Mix eggs with carrot, coconut cream, and liquid honey.
2. Transfer the mixture in the baking cups and bake at 365F for 25 minutes.

NUTRITION: 170 calories, 6.7g protein, 11.7g carbohydrates, 11.5g fat, 2g fiber, 164mg cholesterol, 104mg sodium, 316mg potassium

144. Baked Bananas

Preparation time: 10 minutes

Cooking time: 15 minutes

Servings: 6

INGREDIENTS:

- 6 bananas, halved
- 1 teaspoon ground cinnamon
- 1 teaspoon vanilla extract
- 1 tablespoon almond butter

DIRECTIONS:

1. Rub the banana halves with ground cinnamon, vanilla extract, and almond butter.
2. Put the bananas in the tray and bake at 365F for 15 minutes.

NUTRITION: 124 calories, 1.9g protein, 27.9g carbohydrates, 1.9g fat, 3.5g fiber, 0mg cholesterol, 1mg sodium, 445mg potassium

145. Pomegranate Pudding

Preparation time: 10 minutes

Cooking time: 20 minutes

Servings: 4

INGREDIENTS:

- 1 cup oatmeal
- 2 cups of coconut milk
- 3 almond butter
- ½ cup pomegranate seeds

DIRECTIONS:

1. Bring the coconut milk to boil.
2. Add oatmeal and almond butter.

3. Simmer the mixture for 5 minutes.
4. Then remove it from the heat, add pomegranate seeds and stir well.
5. Transfer the pudding in the serving bowls.

NUTRITION: 440 calories, 8.1g protein, 25.7g carbohydrates, 36.7g fat, 6g fiber, 0mg cholesterol, 20mg sodium, 480mg potassium

146. Mango Pudding

Preparation time: 10 minutes

Cooking time: 0 minutes

Servings: 2

INGREDIENTS:

- 1 mango, peeled, blended
- 1 cup plain yogurt
- 3 oz chia seeds
- 1 teaspoon fresh mint

DIRECTIONS:

1. Mix plain yogurt with chia seeds and put in the serving glasses.
2. Top the yogurt with fresh mint and blended mango.

NUTRITION: 395 calories, 15.4g protein, 51.8g carbohydrates, 15.2g fat, 17.4g fiber, 7mg cholesterol, 95mg sodium, 746mg potassium

147. Matcha Pudding

Preparation time: 10 minutes

Cooking time: 10 minutes

Servings: 4

INGREDIENTS:

- 1 teaspoon matcha powder
- 1 cup coconut cream
- 2 oz chia seeds
- 1 tablespoon liquid honey

DIRECTIONS:

1. Mix matcha powder with coconut cream and bring to boil.

2. Then cool the mixture, add chia seeds and liquid honey.
3. Stir the pudding well.

NUTRITION: 224 calories, 4g protein, 13.6g carbohydrates, 18.7g fat, 6.5g fiber, 0mg cholesterol, 11mg sodium, 225mg potassium

148. Pineapple Sorbet

Preparation time: 50 minutes

Cooking time: 0 minutes

Servings: 4

INGREDIENTS:

- 2 tablespoons of liquid honey
- 1 teaspoon fresh mint
- 2 cups pineapple, chopped

DIRECTIONS:

1. Blend the pineapple until smooth.
2. Add liquid honey and mint. Stir the mixture.
3. Put the mixture in the silicone molds and freeze for 40 minutes.
4. Then remove the mixture from the molds, transfer in the food processor and blend until smooth.
5. Put the dessert in the serving bowls.

NUTRITION: 73 calories, 0.5g protein, 19.5g carbohydrates, 0.1g fat, 1.2g fiber, 0mg cholesterol, 2mg sodium, 98mg potassium

149. Cinnamon Brown Rice Pudding

Preparation time: 10 minutes

Cooking time: 20 minutes

Servings: 5

INGREDIENTS:

- 3 cups of coconut milk
- 1 cup of brown rice
- 1 tablespoon liquid honey
- 1 teaspoon cinnamon powder

DIRECTIONS:

1. Mix coconut milk with brown rice and ground cinnamon.
2. Simmer the mixture for 20 minutes on low heat.
3. Then remove the pudding from the heat, cool little, add liquid honey, and stir the pudding well.

NUTRITION: 482 calories, 6.2g protein, 40.4g carbohydrates, 35.4g fat, 4.5g fiber, 0mg cholesterol, 23mg sodium, 483mg potassium

150. Pumpkin Balls

Preparation time: 10 minutes

Cooking time: 0 minutes

Servings: 4

INGREDIENTS:

- 4 oz pumpkin seeds, crushed
- 1 oz chia seeds
- 5 dates, chopped
- 1 teaspoon honey

DIRECTIONS:

1. Put all ingredients in the mixing bowl and mix until smooth.
2. Make the small balls from the mixture and store them in the fridge for up to 4 days.

NUTRITION: 222 calories, 8.4g protein, 17.3g carbohydrates, 15.2g fat, 4.4g fiber, 0mg cholesterol, 7mg sodium, 327mg potassium

CONCLUSION

Congratulations! You have made it to the end of the Anti-Inflammatory Diet Cookbook. I hope it has benefited you as much as it has benefited me. I enjoyed writing each chapter for you. I included a little bit of everything in this book for the readers' and my information, and enjoyment. Each chapter I created is based on one principle. The same principle is truly a life-altering element to any anti-inflammatory diet. In sharing with you many of the changes I have made in my own diet, I hope that you choose to be inspired and learn to incorporate the anti-inflammatory principles in your own daily life.

Inflammation hurts—there is no way around that particular fact. Inflammation is no fun for anyone that suffers from it and the best cure is prevention. That's where this book comes in—so keep on the path!

I hope you enjoy each and every recipe in this book. Cook with passion and purpose, and always remember that foods not make up a diet. Your diet is made up of the choices you make about what foods you eat, how you cook them, and the meal presentation.

It is my life's work to keep learning about the benefits of an anti-inflammatory diet and healing my body of chronic inflammation. I am a work in progress on the journey to wellness—not arriving—just taking each step as it comes to live in the moment and be grateful for what I have.

I wish you a long life filled with fun, adventure, love, and joy!

Health and Happiness

CPSIA information can be obtained
at www.ICGtesting.com
Printed in the USA
BVHW011508010321
601386BV00012B/891